MASTERCLASS GUIDES

Dr. V's 11 Life Lessons to Help You Weigh Less, Fear Less, and Be More

Duc Vuong, M.D.

ISBN-13: 978-0578403830

ISBN-10: 0578403838

Published by HappyStance Publishing.

Interior formatting and cover design by Tony Loton of LOTONtech Limited, www.lotontech.com.

The information contained in this book is not designed to replace or take the place of any form of medicine or professional medical advice. The information in this book has been provided for educational and entertainment purposes only. The information contained in this book has been compiled from sources deemed reliable, and it is accurate to the best of the Author's knowledge; however, the Author cannot guarantee its accuracy and validity and cannot be held liable for any errors or omissions. Changes are periodically made to this book. You must consult your doctor or get professional medical advice before using any of the suggested remedies, techniques, or information in this book. Upon using the information contained in this book, you agree to hold harmless the Author from and against any damages, costs, and expenses, including any legal fees potentially resulting from the application of any of the information provided by this guide. This disclaimer applies to any damages or injury caused by the use and application, whether directly or indirectly, of any advice or information presented, whether for breach of contract, tort, negligence, personal injury, criminal intent, or under any other cause of action. You agree to accept all risks of using the information presented inside this book. You need to consult a professional medical practitioner in order to ensure you are both able and healthy enough to participate in this program. Although Dr. Vuong is a medical doctor, he is most likely not your doctor, and this book in no way creates a doctor-patient relationship between you, the reader, and him.

Contents

To my two beautiful daughters, Chloe Ann and Maysen Marie.

Always choose kind.

Introduction

In early 2018 I had the realization that if reading books is going the way of television, MySpace, and the dodo bird, then I'd better give people something other than long narrative to help change their lives. But in our hectic world of head-down and swipe-up, what medium could I use to capture and HOLD the attention of my audience?

Then it occurred to me: people want (and need) easily accessible information that can be consumed quickly and is interesting to look at. So I created short, graphic, downloadable PDF reports that were not only useful but also beautiful. And people loved them! These "Dr. V PDFs" became very popular, receiving thousands of downloads. I encouraged people to print them out and create a binder with them. But I soon discovered a problem.

After printing only 2 of the PDFs myself, my printer ran out of ink! The reports were so graphic and colorful that they used up a lot of ink. I really wanted people to have the beauty of these reports all in one place, so I created *this compendium* of my masterclasses.

While this collection of popular PDFs is geared towards the weight loss community, many of the concepts and teachings are applicable to everyone. The topics range from the proper diet to breaking bad habits to saving money, and even how to deal with criticism.

My goal is to have this book become a quick go-to reference and fun read for anyone looking for guidance on the most common questions we encounter in our everyday lives.

All the best,

Dr. Vuong

MASTERCLASS 1
The Dr. V Diet

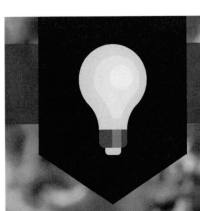

DR V MASTERCLASS PRESENTS

THE DR. V DIET

LIVING YOUR BEST LIFE
WITH GOOD NUTRITION

Prepared by: Dr. Duc Vuong

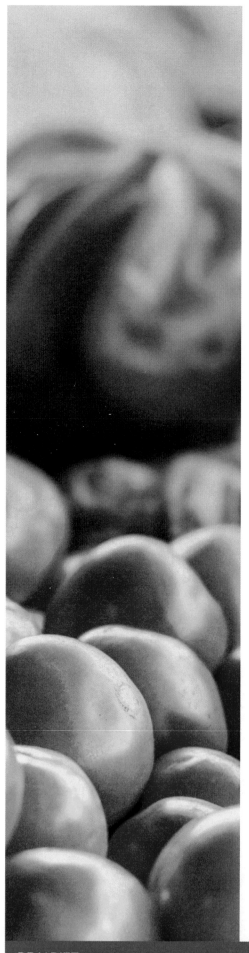

GOOD HEALTH STARTS WITH GOOD FOOD

We eat in order to live. Food supplies us with the calories and building blocks we need to function and to repair our bodies. However, not all food is created equal. Most foods made for our fast paced convenience culture have no nutritional content whatsoever.

In order to live your best life, you need to give your body the right fuel. Today we are going to go over a very simple plan that will ensure you get the nutrition you need and still lose the extra weight. This includes the extra guidelines Post-op patients will need to follow to accommodate their new surgeries.

There is no calorie counting. No severe restrictions. No special secrets or complicated measuring. It is all about making healthy decisions easier with a simple routine.

We'll go over the simple guidelines, a few things to keep in mind for each, and how to customize the experience post-op.

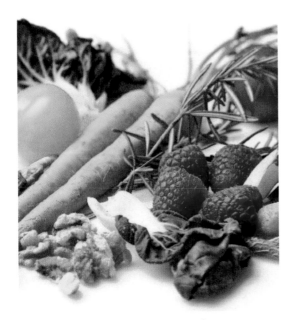

50% Raw Diet

When we say 'raw,' we are talking produce. Fresh and unprocessed fruits and vegetables. This would be your fresh salads, your frozen fruits, and most importantly, your leafy greens.

Plants hold a host of nutrition in them. For example, a serving of spinach is an excellent source of plant protein, Vitamin A, calcium, iron, potassium, and about a dozen other vital nutrients [1].

However, many nutrients are fragile. They will break down and diminish in the process of cooking. So to get the best nutrition, you need to eat them fresh.

There are a lot of benefits aside from just eating healthier. Fresh leafy greens are filling and are very low in calories. Each one is packed with the building blocks you need to perform at home and work at your peak.

These nutrients also help you reduce medical complications too. Studies have shown vegan and raw food diets lower the risk of problems like heart disease and fibromyalgia [2][3].

"But Dr.V, that sounds hard!"

It's super easy, I assure you. The only measuring you need to do is to account for your portion sizes (pre-op or post-op) and make sure you get in a good variety each day.

"If you follow this easy diet, then at least 66% of your diet will be raw foods daily."

YOUR DR. V DIET PLAN

I make it a point not to tell my patients to do anything that I would not do myself. The guideline here is what I also follow every day. Note that 2 out of 3 meals center around raw produce- well over half your total food intake.

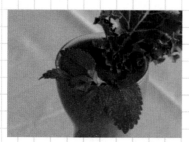

BREAKFAST: ONE GREEN SMOOTHIE

29 out of 30 days, your breakfast should consist of a smoothie of frozen fruits and leafy greens.

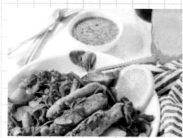

LUNCH: A BIG-ASS SALAD

A variety of leafy greens as the star, topped with veggies, berries, lean proteins, or other healthy toppings.

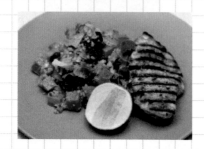

DINNER: ANYTHING (WITHIN REASON)

Anything of reasonable nutritional value and portion size. Skip Dessert. **If you could not get your salad for lunch, do the Big-Ass Salad for dinner.

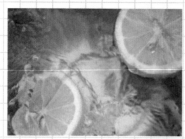

SIP LOTS OF WATER

At least 64 oz of water (four store-bought bottles for perspective)- but aim to sip 80oz or more a day.

NO SNACKING- Unless you are doing a strenuous activity and need to refuel. Snacking is a temptation into old bad habits.

GREEN SMOOTHIES ARE THE HEALTHIEST BREAKFAST POSSIBLE

Despite the name, green smoothies are not green- in fact, my blueberry ones look brown. The name comes from the fact that they are packed with *leafy green* vegetables.

As we discussed before, leafy greens and the accompanying fruits and vegetables all have a host of extra nutrients that you will not find in bacon or a breakfast burrito. In addition, it is already broken down for easy digestion.

To make a basic green smoothie you need:

- A couple handfuls of leafy greens, like spinach
- Some frozen fruits and/or berries
- A banana or avocado will make it creamy if desired
- A liquid base. I use soy milk, though plant-based fluids like coconut milk, almond milk, etc work too.
- Avoid dairy and protein shakes
- No Artificial sweeteners. You might elect for a natural sweetener like honey or agave if desired.

YOU NEED AN EMULSIFIER, NOT A BLENDER!

A regular blender will not create the smoothie texture or break down the nutrients for you efficiently. You'll be making smoothies daily, so opting for a good emulsifier will be a good investment. I use a NutriNinja, which runs around $70- $100, and I have used it daily for a year and a half. Compare that to the money spent on shoes and clothing that is only worn a day or two a month.

You can find my book on 50 Green Smoothie recipes on Amazon.

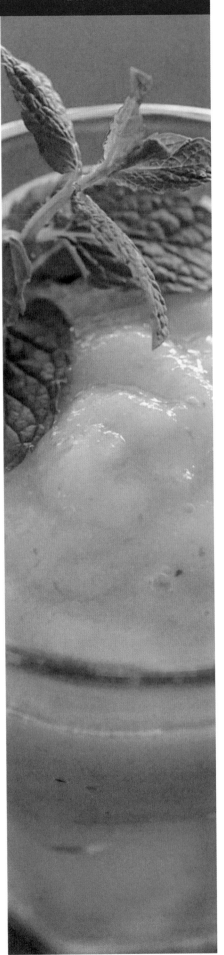

THE BIG-ASS SALAD

Don't think iceberg lettuce with minced carrots. A salad can be a very nutritious, filling and delicious meal if done right!

- Make sure leafy greens are the star of the salad. It should be the most plentiful part of the meal.

- Top it with fresh raw vegetables, fruits, nuts, berries and other toppings for extra taste and nutrition. But make sure they do not overshadow the leafy greens.

- You can even add a little lean meat protein like salmon or shrimp.

- A small amount of cooked foods like quinoa, roasted sweet potatoes, and steamed asparagus can help toss in a little more variety.

- POST-OP: The "Little Big-Ass Salad." You can have a full hand serving of salad because it will squish down in your pouch. Be very mindful of serving size when adding denser toppings.

Need more inspiration? I have a whole month of Dr. V approved Salad recipes to help you get started or shake up your current line-up.

A REASONABLE DINNER

Food is the building material you use to maintain your body. So while you have no true limits on your meal, you should maintain portion control and choose foods that build your body toward your health goals.

Anything

Post-Op is encouraged to stick to level 3 and 4 texture foods, and your pouch can only handle a meal the size of your palm. Otherwise, you have a lot of freedom for dinner.

Don't counteract all the effort you made through the day with a large portion of fatty foods. However, you do have a lot of freedom in this meal given you already got almost all your nutrition from your smoothie and salad.

Reasonable

If it's your kid's birthday, don't beat yourself up over a small slice of pizza. Just don't make those unhealthy moments a habit. Opt for the healthiest options available every day you can.

The vast majority of your meals should supplement the healthy choices you made through the day, like fish for healthy fats.

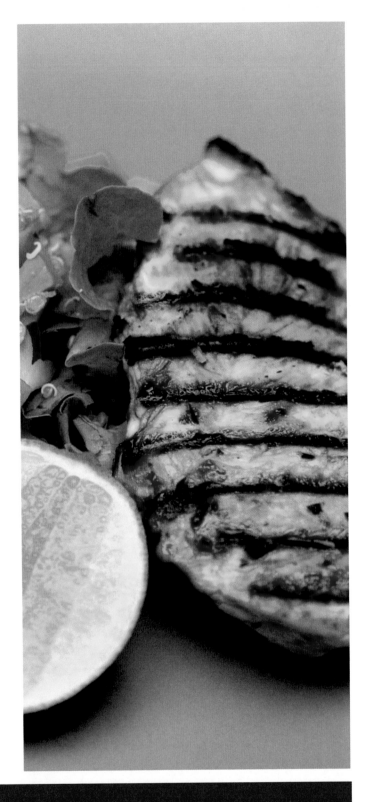

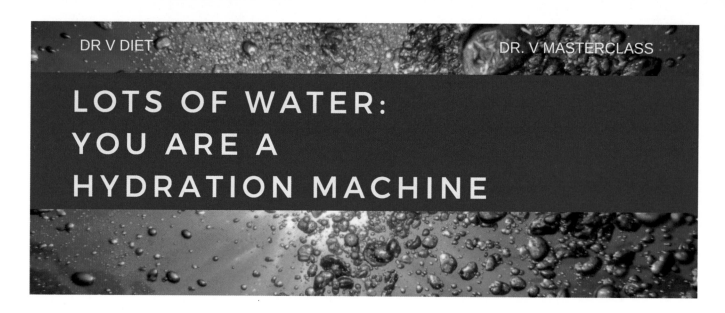

LOTS OF WATER: YOU ARE A HYDRATION MACHINE

Water is an often overlooked part of your nutrition, but it is also one of the most vital. You could live weeks, maybe even months, on your own body fat. However, your organs start shutting down after only a few days without water. Even a low amount of dehydration can cause mind fog and fatigue. Severe dehydration can even cause you very serious health problems like seizures, fainting, and organ damage [4].

Note we are talking water. Not sugary fruit drinks, sodas, teas, or coffees. These are liquid forms of empty calories that just put more work on your digestive system. A few ways to hit your daily goal of 80 oz are:

- Start AND end your day. Have a glass of water handy by your bed when you wake up and go to sleep.
- Use Kangen water if you can afford it. I own a machine and love it.
- Get a good filter. I personally recommend Zero Water filters. I found after a personal test that it does indeed clear out all the silt and contaminants other filters miss.
- Infusing water with fresh fruit or cucumbers will help if you have trouble moving from flavored beverages to pure water. Use the leftover fruits in your green smoothies.
- Get a large marked jug that lets you compare the water level and see if you are falling short of your goal.

POST OP: DEHYDRATION IS THE TOP REASON FOR READMISSION INTO THE HOSPITAL [5]

Your pouch cannot handle you 'catching up' by chugging a bottle of water. Consider alarms and apps that will remind you to take a couple sips every 15 minutes until it becomes a set habit.

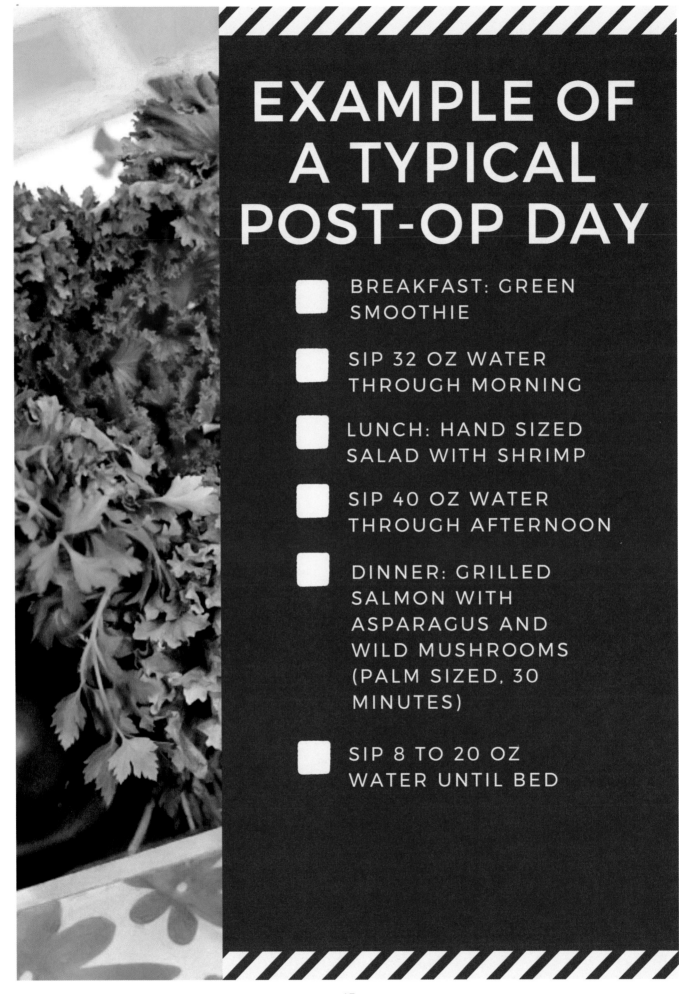

EXAMPLE OF A TYPICAL POST-OP DAY

- [ ] BREAKFAST: GREEN SMOOTHIE

- [ ] SIP 32 OZ WATER THROUGH MORNING

- [ ] LUNCH: HAND SIZED SALAD WITH SHRIMP

- [ ] SIP 40 OZ WATER THROUGH AFTERNOON

- [ ] DINNER: GRILLED SALMON WITH ASPARAGUS AND WILD MUSHROOMS (PALM SIZED, 30 MINUTES)

- [ ] SIP 8 TO 20 OZ WATER UNTIL BED

LISTEN TO YOUR BABY

Eat slowly, and when you feel pressure- STOP.

ACCEPT THE CONSEQUENCES

If you eat after you are full, snack, or make unhealthy choices--be prepared to accept the UNDESIRED results.

PARTING THOUGHTS

Good nutrition does not have to be hard. Nor does it have to be restricting. If you follow these guidelines, you will feel healthier. You will lose excess weight.

Plus you will have a lot more freedom to have many foods you thought you would have to give up.

Green Smoothie
Big Ass Salad
A Reasonable Dinner
80 oz Water
No Snacking

This is the simple DR. V DIET formula that will help you achieve your weight and health goals.

WEEKLY
MEAL PLAN

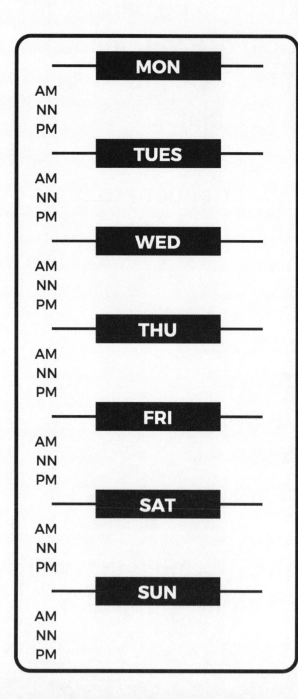

MON

AM
NN
PM

TUES

AM
NN
PM

WED

AM
NN
PM

THU

AM
NN
PM

FRI

AM
NN
PM

SAT

AM
NN
PM

SUN

AM
NN
PM

THINGS TO BUY

NOTES:

[1] Spinach, Raw Nutrition Facts & Calories . (2018). Nutritiondata.self.com. Retrieved 9 August 2018, from http://nutritiondata.self.com/facts/vegetables-and-vegetable-products/2626/2

[2] Donaldson, M. S., Speight, N., & Loomis, S. (2001). Fibromyalgia syndrome improved using a mostly raw vegetarian diet: an observational study. BMC complementary and alternative medicine, 1(1), 7.

[3] Hu F. B. Plant-based foods and prevention of cardiovascular disease: an overview. Am. J. Clin. Nutr. 2003;78:544S–551S.

[4] Dehydration - Symptoms and causes. (2018). Mayo Clinic. Retrieved 27 July 2018, from https://www.mayoclinic.org/diseases-conditions/dehydration/symptoms-causes/syc-20354086

[5] Life After Bariatric Surgery | American Society for Metabolic and Bariatric Surgery. (2018). American Society for Metabolic and Bariatric Surgery. Retrieved 27 July 2018, from https://asmbs.org/patients/life-after-bariatric-surgery

MASTERCLASS 2

Hospital Stay

HOSPITAL STAY

3 CRITICAL THINGS YOU MUST DO AFTER SURGERY

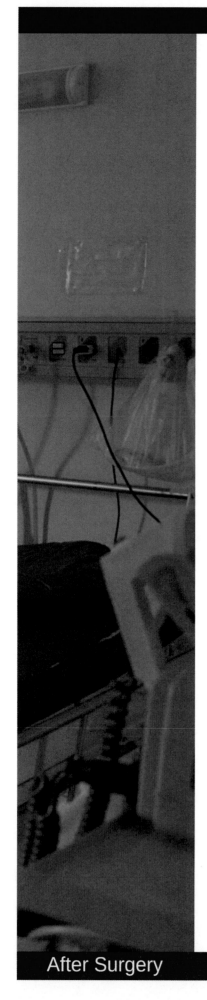

Introduction

Of all your friends and family who qualify for weight loss surgery, only about 1% will actually have the courage to go through with it.

Congratulations on taking your health seriously enough to begin preparing for what happens after surgery! You are well on your way to beating the odds.

Don't rest on your laurels yet. Weight loss surgery will only mark the start of a new chapter in your journey. We are going to cover a few things you should plan to do directly after surgery that will reduce serious complications and build a good foundation for the next chapter of your journey.

These three postoperative requirements are deceptively simple, but they are essential for the prevention of complications after surgery:

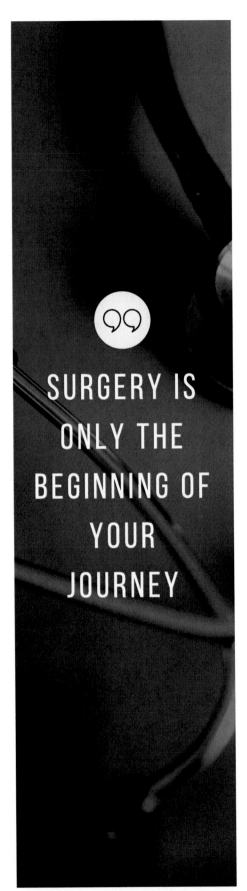

SURGERY IS ONLY THE BEGINNING OF YOUR JOURNEY

3 ESSENTIAL THINGS TO DO AFTER SURGERY

1. WALK

Within hours of surgery, most will be asked to begin walking for short periods. The frequency and distance will persist even after you leave the hospital.

2. SIP, SIP, SIP

The day of your surgery, you will most likely not be given any fluids. The next day you will start out on ice chips. Variability exists among different programs, but regardless of the program you choose, you will be spending the rest of your life as a water sipping machine.

3. BREATHE

As soon as you are alert enough, you will be introduced to a device called an incentive spirometer. You will use it hourly to open and strengthen your lungs even after you return home from surgery.

1. WALKING IT OUT

While there are many important health benefits to walking, the primary reason your healthcare team will push you to start moving around and walking is to reduce the risk of blood clots [1].

Any surgery carries a risk of developing an abnormal clot. Deep vein thrombosis (DVT) can occur in the veins, particularly in the lower legs. In rare occasions, the clot can break off and travel to the lungs, restricting appropriate oxygen exchange. This is called a pulmonary embolism, or PE for short. Movement helps reduce the risk of clot formation [2][3].

As soon as the nurses feel you can move out of bed safely, expect them to assist you in walking around. No old-lady shuffles--use your legs and walk as naturally as you can to promote proper blood circulation. Use proper handholds for stability. If you are able, throw in some toe lifts and calf raises for good measure.

Walking also provides long-term benefits as well [1], such as:

- Improved immune system
- Reduced appetite (in short sessions)
- Reduction in minor fatigue and sluggishness.
- Improved balance as your body shape changes
- Increased overall sense of wellbeing

Walking After Surgery

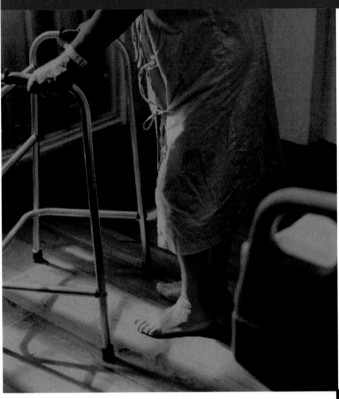

IN THE HOSPITAL

Each person is different, but in general, you can expect to begin short bursts of walking and physical therapy within hours of surgery. Listen to your nurses and physical therapists. If they tell you it's time to walk, don't wave them off. GET UP AND GO!

DO NOT SHUFFLE. You will not promote good blood circulation with a penguin walk. Add in some calf raises if you can.

AT HOME

Take it slow at first. Walk 5 times a day in short bursts. Increase the distance and duration as you heal, eventually walking every hour.

Wear comfortable and secure footwear to make sure you don't slip or fall.

In the early days, make sure you walk where you have secure handholds.

Don't hurt yourself falling. Avoid loose rugs and slick or uneven surfaces at home or outside.

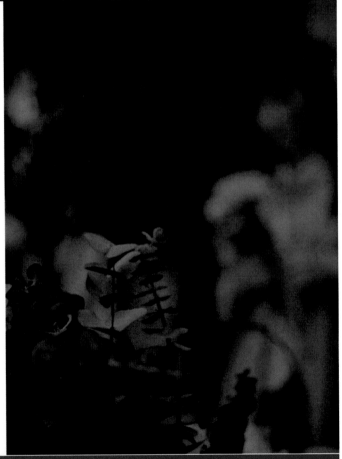

After Surgery

Dr V Masterclass

2. Sip, Sip, Sip!

The first day, your medical team most likely will keep your mouth dry as your body recovers from surgery. Don't worry, you will be receiving fluids through your IV. Then you will graduate to ice chips, then sips of water. Fluid intake will be one of your most important challenges.

Dehydration is a common reason for readmission to the hospital [4] after weight loss surgery. This is because many patients--as they are recovering from surgery, waking from anesthesia, dealing with pain-- are not mindful of their fluid intake as they adjust to their new pouch.

Dehydration causes a host of medical issues. Lack of proper fluids keeps the liver and kidneys from functioning at optimal levels. Blood volume thickens and makes it harder to deliver nutrients and oxygen around the body. It can even cause shock, blood clot formation, and seizures [5].

You will not have space in your pouch to gulp down large amounts of fluids at once, so sipping all day and every day will be your new obsession. You will have to keep close track of how much you take in to ensure you hydrate properly.

In the meantime, you will also have to retrain your brain. Instead of being obsessed with food, water becomes your new addiction.

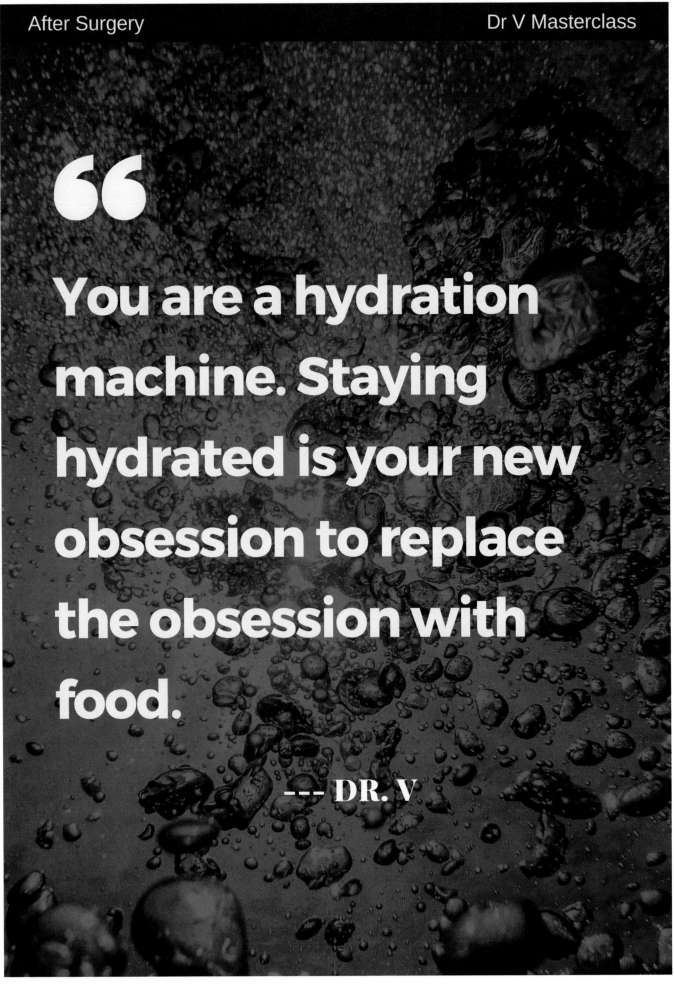

You are a hydration machine. Staying hydrated is your new obsession to replace the obsession with food.

--- DR. V

SIP TIPS

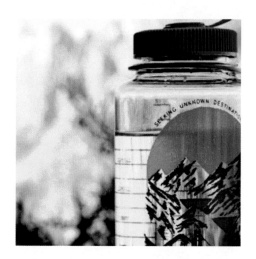

64 oz of water is the absolute minimum you should aim for. But this will be very difficult the first couple of days after surgery. That is four 16 oz bottles of water from the store for perspective. Ideally you should drink closer to 80 oz daily.

Make sure to drink immediately after waking up, to get your body started for the day. Keeping a glass of water where you will see and reach for it when you wake up can help with this.

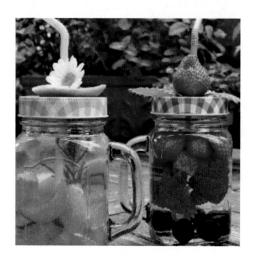

There are various apps out there that will let you set alarms and track your hydration effortlessly.

Do not substitute water with soda, sugary fruit juices, or other drinks. Instead you can infuse water with fresh fruits, but remember to NOT EAT the leftover fruit. Stick to low acid fruits in the beginning while you adjust to your surgery.

Drink tea in moderation. Most teas are diuretics, and too much can lead to dehydration. Do not add calories with creamers or sweeteners. **Avoid coffee during this period.**

FOOD FOR THOUGHT

You can live up to 8 weeks without food but only 3-5 days without water.

SIP! You do not want to make yourself sick by gulping down your water. You don't have a lot of pouch room to rush hydration. From now on

YOU ARE A HYDRATION MACHINE

3. Breathe

While you can go weeks without food and a few days without water, you can only go a few minutes without air. Even a small drop in the oxygen concentration in your blood can cause increased fatigue and confusion. **So take your breathing seriously.**

Because you just had a major surgery which required intubation anesthesia, the air sacs in your lungs collapse and they stick together like the inside of a water balloon once it is emptied--a condition called atelectasis [6]. This is further exasperated by lying in bed during recuperation.

After surgery, you have to open these air sacs. You will be given a machine called an incentive spirometer to help with this task. You'll suck in air as hard as you can through the device in order to pop these deflated sacs back open and promote better oxygen intake.

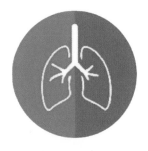

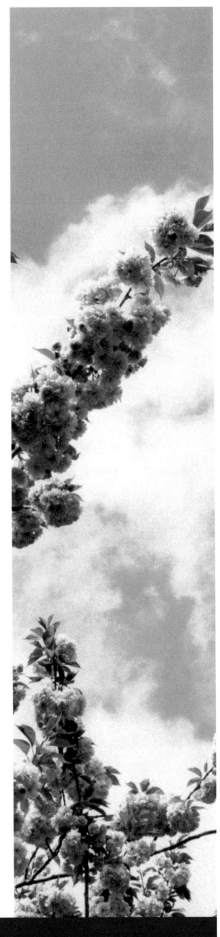

BREATHING TIPS

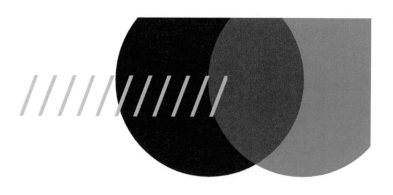

01 SUCK, DON'T BLOW

Many surgery patients will start out trying to blow into the machine. Don't be one of them. The Spirometer is made to help you open your lungs. This is accomplished by deeply inhaling, not exhaling.

02 OPEN THOSE LUNGS

When you receive your spirometer, you will be told to suck in just hard enough to hover the ball inside between two marks- IGNORE THAT. Between years of obesity and the recent surgery, you gotta pop open those air sacs. Suck as hard and long as you can every hour.

03 KEEP DOING IT AT HOME

Don't let up on this when you get home. Set your calendars and alarms to remind you to do your breathing exercises. When your doctor says you can stop the spirometer, switch to deep breathing exercises.

04 BE PREPARED

It's going to hurt, and you are going to cough up goop. Keep pushing forward. Once your lungs strengthen and clear themselves out, this sucking exercise will get easier.

05 MIND YOUR ENVIROMENT

Don't forget that things like air quality, allergies, smoking, and air pollution are still factors in your lung health after surgery [7].

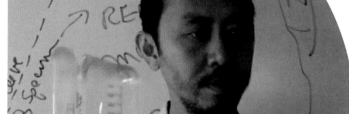

These three simple measures make a HUGE impact on your continued journey.

You've made it this far! Make sure your post-surgery experience is just as successful.

Walk those legs.
Sip that water.
Suck on that machine.

Keep fighting for that healthy life you dreamed about.

YOU CAN DO IT!

PERSONAL TRACKER

Date today:

Water:

_____

_____

_____

_____

_____

_____

_____

_____

_____

Walking:

_____

_____

_____

Breathing:

_____

_____

_____

RECORD THE TIMES AND AMOUNTS OR
DURATION TO TRACK YOUR PROGRESS

[1] How to Prevent Blood Clots After Surgery. (2018). Healthline. Retrieved 27 July 2018, from https://www.healthline.com/health/how-to-prevent-blood-clots-after-surgery

[2] Bariatric Surgery: Postoperative Concerns | American Society for Metabolic and Bariatric Surgery. (2018). American Society for Metabolic and Bariatric Surgery. Retrieved 27 July 2018, from https://asmbs.org/resources/bariatric-surgery-postoperative-concerns-2

[3]Blood Clots. (2018). Hematology.org. Retrieved 27 July 2018, from http://www.hematology.org/Patients/Clots/

[4]Life After Bariatric Surgery | American Society for Metabolic and Bariatric Surgery. (2018). American Society for Metabolic and Bariatric Surgery. Retrieved 27 July 2018, from https://asmbs.org/patients/life-after-bariatric-surgery

[5] Dehydration - Symptoms and causes. (2018). Mayo Clinic. Retrieved 27 July 2018, from https://www.mayoclinic.org/diseases-conditions/dehydration/symptoms-causes/syc-20354086

[6] https://www.healthpages.org/surgical-care/preventing-lung-problems-after-surgery-general-anesthesia/

[7] Raveendran Nair, M. Atmospheric Pollution and Lung Health. Radiology Quiz, 99.

MASTERCLASS 3
The First Month After Surgery

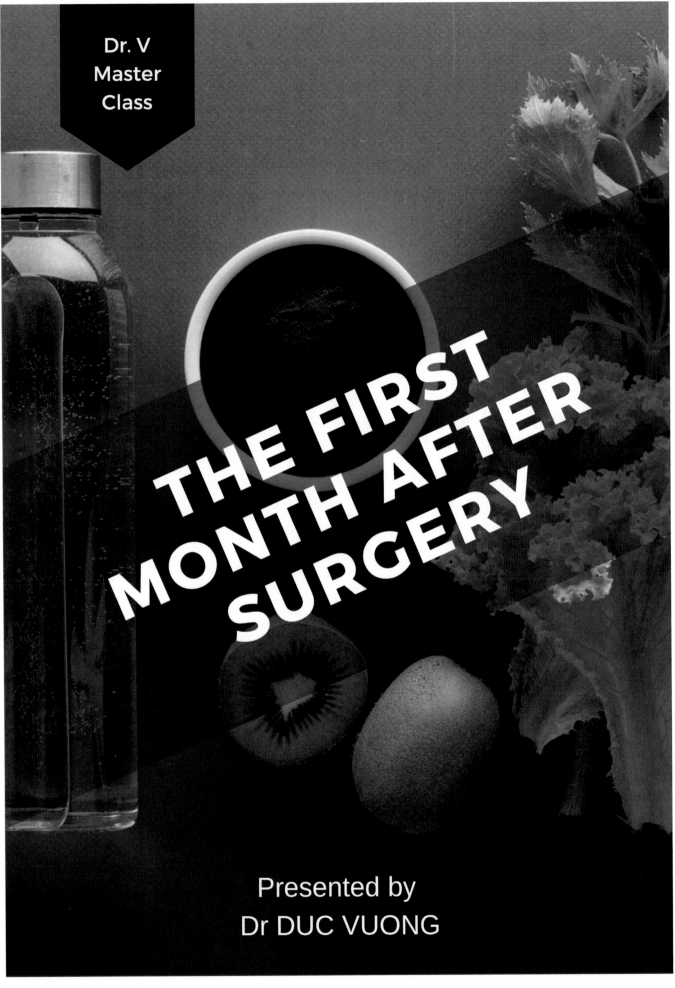

Dr. V
Master
Class

THE FIRST MONTH AFTER SURGERY

Presented by
Dr DUC VUONG

IT'S TIME FOR A NEW CHAPTER IN YOUR LIFE

Congratulations!

You've done all the work. You made all your preparations. Now the post-surgery phase of your journey is here.

And it is going to be a roller coaster.

It will be rewarding, but your "minimally invasive" surgery is still **major** surgery. It is going to create some massive changes in your life. And like all massive changes, you have that exciting yet uncomfortable adjustment phase.

Today we're going to cover some of the major things to expect in the first month after surgery. The very first thing you need to really let sink in is-

YOU JUST HAD MAJOR SURGERY

You have a few small scars, and you were moving around within hours of surgery. And it wasn't long before you made your way home. It can be easy to overlook exactly how drastic a change you just underwent.

But these things do not change the fact **you just had major surgery**, and that you have undergone significant changes on the inside, namely your much smaller stomach capacity.

This means you have a long way to go in the actual recovery process. Treat yourself and your new surgery with great care, and be patient with the process. There is no need to try to rush your healing or jump back to all your work and other responsibilities right away. Rushing back into life is a COMMON MISTAKE patients often make.

THINGS TO REMEMBER IN THE HOSPITAL:

The nurses are going to start you on walking and moving as soon as you are able. This is to avoid blood clots and other medical issues [1], so don't turn them away.

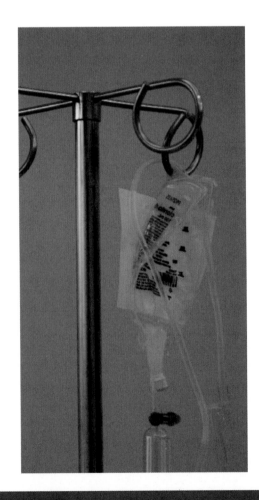

You most likely won't be given oral liquids the first day. You'll receive the fluids you need through an IV. Once you get the okay for water, sip-sip-sip! Hydration is now you new biggest challenge and obsession.

Take things slowly. Don't try to rush your healing process. If you do, you'll feel like crap and gain very little reward for it.

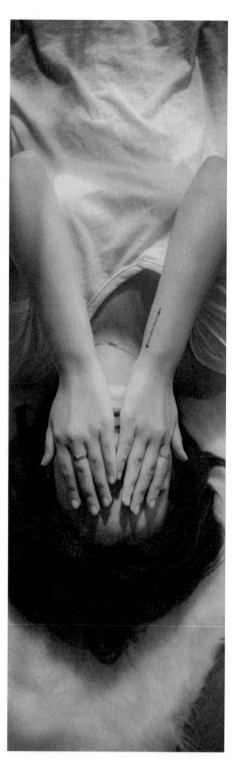

What The Fudge?

Pre-op you were excited and full of energy. Anticipation was high. You will continue to ride that excitement wave the first few days after surgery.

Post-surgery the reality kicks in. You're exhausted from the sudden drop in calories. Everything aches. You are still adapting to proper hydration and how slowly you need to consume everything.

While you most likely won't experience physical hunger, you will feel withdrawal from the habit of eating. You might even begin to feel buyer's remorse for putting yourself through this. **THE WHOLE PROCESS MIGHT FEEL OVERWHELMING.**

Like a new baby, your new stomach has turned habits and routines and comfort zones into chaos. Adjusting to this new reality will take time.

For most of the first month, it is normal to feel tired, frustrated with your body, and even overwhelmed [3]. This is why we always encourage you to take as much time off work and your regular responsibilities as you can afford -- to allow time to adjust to the new "baby."

Your support groups will be vital to help you remember that you are not alone and that this phase is *normal*.

The worst day is usually 5 to 6 days after surgery. The exhaustion from low calories and the surgical pain/swelling catches up to you.
-- Dr. V

NO WEIGHT LOSS

Fluid Fluctuations

High Calories, Low Nutrition in Mushy Stage

Medication Changes

First Month Should Focus on Recovery

You will experience very dramatic weight fluctuations during the first two weeks. In fact, I don't allow my patients to weigh at all the first week because the huge fluid shifts will cause extreme fluctuations in weight.

This first month is about healing, getting used to life with your new stomach, and self development, including getting rid of negative "friends."

After dramatic (and easy) weight loss the first month, you might hit a plateau at the 4-6 week mark. DO NOT BE ALARMED. This is very common! It is due to the reintroduction of food into your diet. Use the first few months to get your routines and new habits in place.

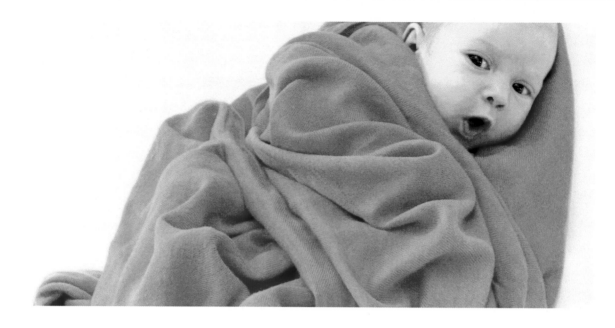

LISTEN TO BABY

Your weight loss surgery is very much like a baby. It is completely dependent on you to be alert and attentive to its needs. It will be content when its needs are attended to. It will fuss and give signs (pressure) when it is at its limit. And it will throw a full tantrum (pain, vomiting, etc) if you ignore the signs or try to push 'baby' to deal with things at *your* desired pace.

Over time, you will learn to recognize when your new stomach is saying it is full. You'll recognize a pressure that says it's too soon to eat certain foods on your food calendar. You'll know if you need to change your eating plans and patterns.

Most importantly--DO NOT push to keep up with any information you received pre-op. By this I mean the food calendar, when you should exercise, when to go to work, are all estimates and averages. Like a baby, your surgery will heal and accustom itself to food at its own pace. YOUR BABY IS UNIQUE!

Your baby sets the pace and schedule. If you listen to the signs, you will have fewer pains and progress at a natural pace for you.

HYDRATION

Your New Obsession

Dehydration is one of the most common reasons for re-admittance to the hospital after surgery [2]. Since you no longer have capacity to gulp water in one sitting, you have to spend your waking hours sipping to get the 64 to 80+ ounces of water a day you need to function at your best. This **hydration habit** will be the new obsession to replace food. Here are a few tips to get you started on the right track:

- Listen to Baby. Even with water, you have a limit to how much and how fast you can drink.
- There will be swelling from surgery the first week. At one point, the available space may only be the size of a pencil tip. If you feel you are physically unable to consume the water you need, talk to your nurses and surgeon so they can make sure things are okay and get you an iv if necessary.
- There are free apps and alarms that you can use to track your water consumption. Once you are ready for water, set alarms to remind you to take a sip every 5 minutes until constant sipping becomes a habit.
- Avoid sugary sodas, store-bought juices, and coffees. These are all empty calories and irritants to your already sensitive stomach lining.
- Buy containers with measurement marks. Then you can physically see if you are falling behind on your hydration.
- Check your pee. If your urine is a light yellow color, you are hydrated. The darker it is, the more dehydrated you are.

FOOD CALENDAR

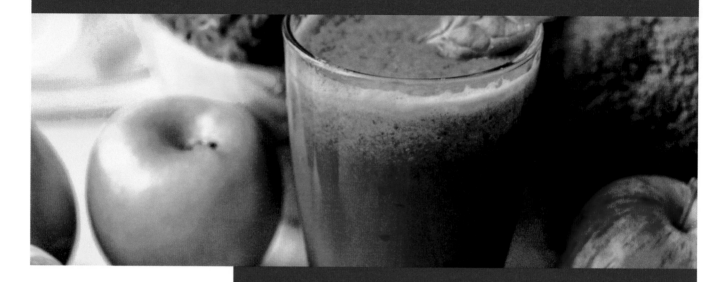

TYPICAL FOOD STAGES

Water Only

Liquids (Enfamil, juice, etc)

Mushy (Green Smoothies, mashed potatoes, etc)

Soft solids (Mashed fruit, fish)

Solids

You'll reintroduce food in stages according to the guidelines your surgeon has provided. Regardless of your program's teachings, don't rush your body to conform to the paperwork you receive. **Everything is an estimate!** So keep in close contact with your medical team. And there will be times your baby handles one stage great one day and backtracks to fluids the next.

With each meal take in a very small taste (ex: with mushy stage, dip your spoon in, then lick the back of it.) Then wait to see how your baby responds. If there is pressure or other signs of pending distress, stop.

It is perfectly fine to progress the food chart slower than it estimates. But never try to rush. You are not in a race or time limit.

Medications

While you are healing, you only have so much space in your pouch to house medicine and the food or fluids required to process them. On top of that, some may irritate the sensitive lining.

Your team will most likely limit your medications to only critical health conditions, such as diabetes, heart, COPD, etc. If the dosage is a large pill, consult your PHARMACIST (before the prescribing doctor) on if you can crush them, move to a liquid form, and alternate, etc. ALWAYS follow the advice of your medical professional.

Also expect to be on an antacid the first few months. You'll most likely also be on pain and anti-nausea medicines post-surgery.

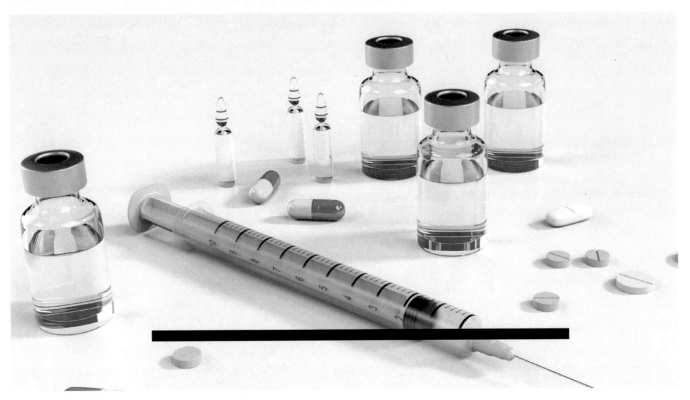

SELF CARE

A weight loss plateau is very common around the 4-6 week mark as you progress through the food calendar. So it is unproductive to put too much emphasis on your weight at this point because it WILL be very frustrating.

Instead, this is the time to focus on yourself. This is the time to establish good habits, to learn meditation and mindfulness exercises. To journal and learn healthy coping skills for stress.

In short, this is your time to rest and work on the foundation of your new life journey.

While you are in this stage, you can be productive in many ways:

- Use the time to rest and learn a new skill.
- Learn a new hobby or enjoy an old one.
- Journal
- Reflect on your long term goals.
- Create a bucket list, with the steps you need to fulfill each one.
- Research ways to budget your healthier lifestyle.
- Contemplate how you will handle your future loose skin.
- Go to your support groups if you find them helpful.
- Get your head on straight: Seek counseling for the things that triggered the over-eating in the first place.
- Subscribe to a self-enrichment program like Rosetta stone, an online class, or a learning app.
- Ask yourself the hard questions about dealing with the rest of the year: relationships, holidays, social situations, etc.

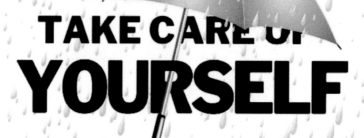

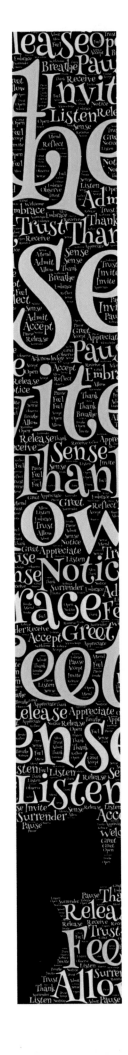

TOUGH QUESTIONS TO CONTEMPLATE

WHAT TRIGGERED MY BAD HABITS IN THE FIRST PLACE? WHAT DO I NEED TO DO IN ORDER TO AVOID A REPEAT?

HOW WILL THIS [HALLOWEEN, CHRISTMAS, ETC] LOOK?

HOW DO I ASK PEOPLE NOT TO SEND RESTAURANT GIFT CARDS AND FOOD GIFTS FOR BIRTHDAYS AND OTHER SPECIAL OCCASIONS?

HOW DO I HANDLE THE PEOPLE WHO TRY TO FORCE FOOD ON ME?

ARE THERE ANY PEOPLE OR EVENTS THAT I NEED TO REMOVE FROM MY LIFE FOR MY PHYSICAL AND EMOTIONAL HEALTH?

WHAT DO I WANT TO DO WITH MY LIFE OVER THE NEXT YEAR?

HOW WILL I HANDLE PLACES PEOPLE EXPECT YOU TO EAT, LIKE A WEDDING OR BIRTHDAY?

HOW WILL I RESPOND TO PEOPLE WHO HEAR ABOUT MY SURGERY?

HOW WILL I RESPOND TO PEOPLE WHO CRITICIZE MY NEW EATING HABITS?

WHAT WILL MY RESPONSE BE IF PEOPLE THINK I AM TAKING TOO LONG TO RECOVER FROM SURGERY? OR IF THEY THINK I AM LOSING WEIGHT TOO SLOWLY?

WHAT WILL BE MY CRITERIA TO KNOW I AM READY TO GO BACK TO WORK? SHOULD I START LOOKING AT NEW EMPLOYMENT OPPORTUNITIES WHILE I AM RECOVERING?

WHAT ONE BIG THING DO I WANT TO ENJOY OR ACCOMPLISH IN THE NEXT YEAR THAT IS 100% FOR MYSELF? WHAT DO I NEED TO DO TO ACCOMPLISH IT?

HOW WILL I ROTATE MY RECIPES AND INGREDIENTS TO MAKE SURE I GET AS MUCH NUTRITION AS POSSIBLE?

You are entering an exciting new chapter in your life. Still, like all new things, it will have its frustrations and overwhelming moments.

Remember that the first month is only the beginning! It's an interlude that marks your latest journey.

Be Mindful.
Be Patient.
Be Ready to Adapt to Challenges
And Most of all

**Love Yourself
and Your New Future**

[1] Dehydration - Symptoms and causes. (2018). Mayo Clinic. Retrieved 27 July 2018, from https://www.mayoclinic.org/diseases-conditions/dehydration/symptoms-causes/syc-20354086

[2] Bariatric Surgery: Postoperative Concerns | American Society for Metabolic and Bariatric Surgery. (2018). American Society for Metabolic and Bariatric Surgery. Retrieved 27 July 2018, from https://asmbs.org/resources/bariatric-surgery-postoperative-concerns-2

[3] Life After Bariatric Surgery | American Society for Metabolic and Bariatric Surgery. (2018). American Society for Metabolic and Bariatric Surgery. Retrieved 27 July 2018, from https://asmbs.org/patients/life-after-bariatric-surgery

MASTERCLASS 4

The Gym is a Punishment

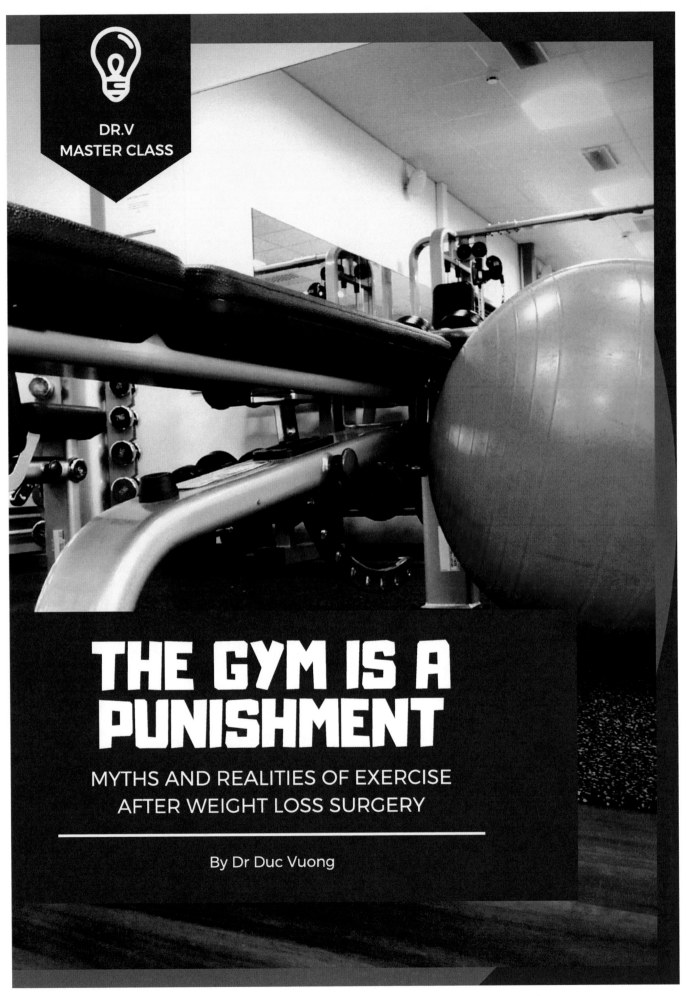

THE GYM IS A PUNISHMENT

MYTHS AND REALITIES OF EXERCISE AFTER WEIGHT LOSS SURGERY

By Dr Duc Vuong

You just had weight loss surgery. You're feeling great. And you are ready and eager to make dramatic changes to your life. You can't wait to finally shed those pounds and get down to an ideal figure. So the next stop is the gym. That's your reward, right? Getting to go work out, lose that weight, and finally get that healthy lifestyle?

Wrong!

I've seen this mistake more times than I can count.

The gym is the worst thing you can do to yourself right after weight loss surgery! In fact, I can guarantee going to the gym right away will sabotage the entire point of your surgery. I know you *really, really, really* want to do what is right, but I promise you are punishing yourself by going about it in the worst way possible. I will explain why in this report.

Before you buy that gym membership, read this report carefully. By the time you are done, you will know 1) why the gym is a punishment rather than a treat, 2) why you should avoid exercise right after weight loss surgery, and most importantly 3) *when and how* you can start exercising again.

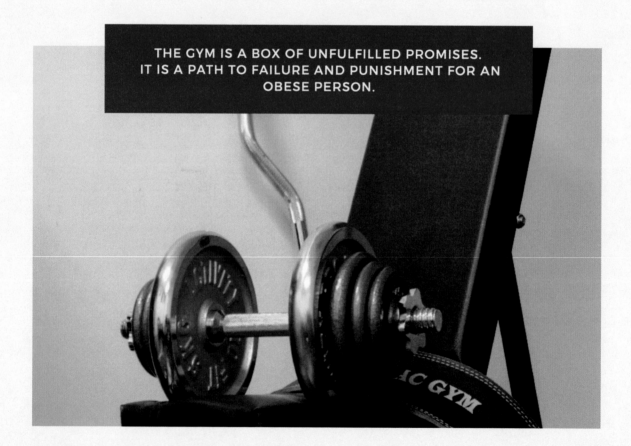

THE GYM IS A BOX OF UNFULFILLED PROMISES.
IT IS A PATH TO FAILURE AND PUNISHMENT FOR AN
OBESE PERSON.

The Gym is a PUNISHMENT

A punishment is a penalty. Its sole purpose is to discourage you from doing something. A punishment makes that course of action painful.

Who would want to go to a gym while morbidly obese? Your regular clothes don't fit. Your gym clothes are uncomfortable. Most have mirrors showing off every move you make from the worst angles you can imagine. You're surrounded by fit, skinny people who are sprinting on the treadmill and bench-pressing weights heavier than they are. The equipment is unfamiliar. **And it feels like all eyes are on you, even if they aren't.**

Then you leave aching, tired, emotionally exhausted, and **hungry**. You feel cravings (you had hoped the surgery would remove) as your body reacts to the sudden activity. You may even give into that hunger and "snack" on something- immediately counteracting all the calories burned at the gym.

Now comes the guilt. If you continue the process, you'll feel tired and discouraged and uncomfortable. If you skip it, you feel like you are failing your weight loss goals. The hunger is back. Many bad eating habits are back. And you are not seeing the results you need to keep you motivated. And this is where many weight loss surgery patients start their slow spiral into undoing everything their surgery was supposed to achieve. In going to the gym to lose weight, it penalizes the efforts instead.

The worst part? Gyms are glorified as the place to go to get fit and lose weight. But it is an empty promise. In actuality-

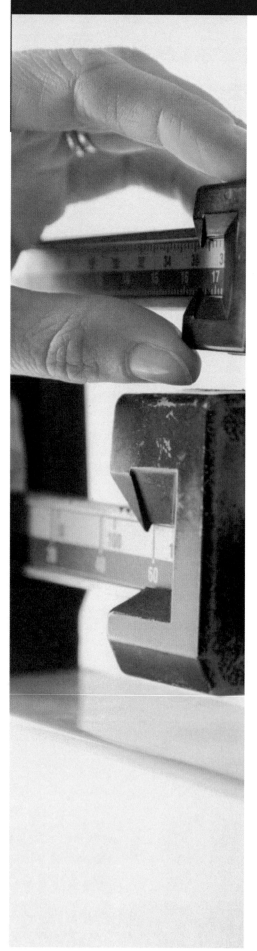

THE GYM DOES NOT HELP YOU LOSE WEIGHT

The gym is not designed for weight loss. Every qualified trainer knows that weight loss starts in the kitchen, not the gym.

This is a Fat-Brain belief that we learn from the ads and a society that glorifies going to the gym as an act of self-love. Healthy people know that the gym will not help them lose weight. It is where they go to build stamina, strengthen heart with cardio, build muscles, and other long-term goals unrelated to their weight.

Let's myth-bust this societal belief right now. Because the sooner you understand why *you can't exercise your way to thin*, the sooner you can focus on more important techniques for your long term success.

Let's say on your first day you got ambitious and brisk-walked two miles on the treadmill. It took "forever." Your calves are burning. You're panting for breath. Sweat is dripping down your back. Heart is thumping. Assuming you were around 300 pounds, you just burned a whopping 349 calories [1]. Good job!

You are exhausted, so you grab a "healthy snack"--a bottle of Gatorade (140 calories, 34 grams sugar) and a protein bar (330 calories, 23 grams sugar). This one snack was MORE calories than what you burned at the gym! Plus you have a simple-sugar crash to deal with on top of the exhaustion.

You CAN'T Exercise Off A Bad Diet

Six More Reasons to Skip the Gym Right After Surgery

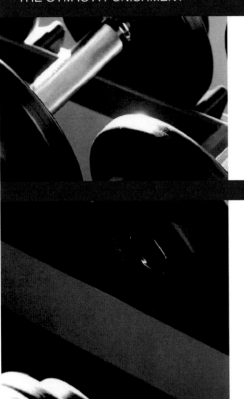

NOT ENOUGH CALORIES

Your recent surgery is designed to restrict the calories you take in. Even if you went to the gym for the right reasons, you would not be able to take in the calories needed to support your bones, muscles and systems through the strain [2].

GUILT AND FAILURE

As you fail to see tangible results in your goals, a cycle of guilt and failure for each skipped gym session and bad food choice will pile on.

NEW HABITS IN PERIL

You need a minimum of 66 days to ingrain a new behavior into a solid habit.[3] If you start exercising right after WLS, the increased hunger will return before you can build your new healthier eating habits. Old habits and cravings will return.

WILL STALL WEIGHT LOSS

The combination of returned cravings, bad habits, and exhaustion will distract from your weight loss goals. At best it will stall the progress you should be making. At worst you will backslide and regain all the weight you lost with the surgery.

HUNGER WILL RETURN

When you suddenly increase activity, your body starts seeking caloried, and it makes a ton of hunger hormones to remind you to refuel. Which means the window of no hunger you wanted to use to get your life back on track has quickly diminished.

EXHAUSTED AND DEMOTIVATED

As all these things come together and escalate. Coupled with the natural fatigue you will feel from increased activity, it will escalate until you burn out and stop trying at all.

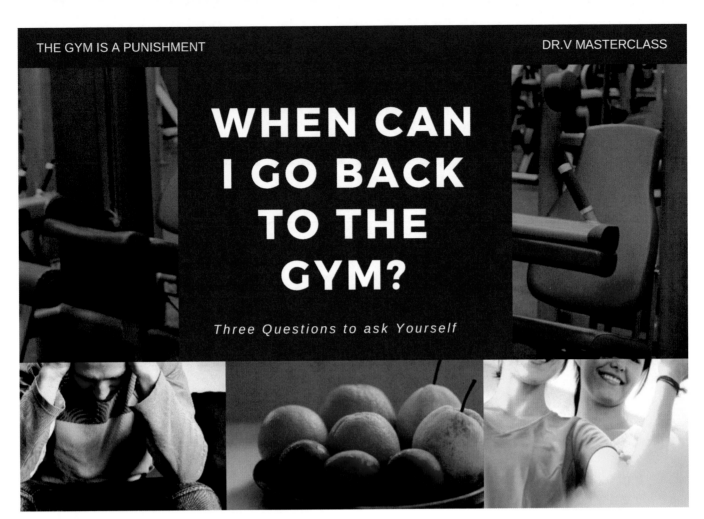

WHEN CAN I GO BACK TO THE GYM?

Three Questions to ask Yourself

IS YOUR HEAD STRAIGHT?

Have you taken care of the things that led to your obesity in the first place? Are you still demotivated by depression? Do marriage problems still cause you significant stress? Do you have healthy coping behaviors for stress?

IS YOUR NUTRITION STRAIGHT?

Are you still stress snacking? Are you drinking your green smoothies? Have you developed solid eating habits that will help you cope with the hunger and physical strain?

CAN YOU AFFORD A PERSONAL TRAINER?

If the answer is no, then you are not ready for the gym. Period. Without proper guidance, you'll waste too much time doing the wrong exercises and risk injury.

These three things together form a triangle of success. Each one reinforces the other two to help you achieve your new goals while protecting your current weight loss and fitness goals. A weakness in one affects all three. Until you have all three straight, the gym is not the place for you.

Without these three factors in place, you will relive a cycle of failure and punishment over and over again. And as we proved earlier: The gym is not a place for weight loss. You need to fix your head, your support, and your dinner plate before you try to tackle the psychological challenges of a gym.

Let's go over each one individually.

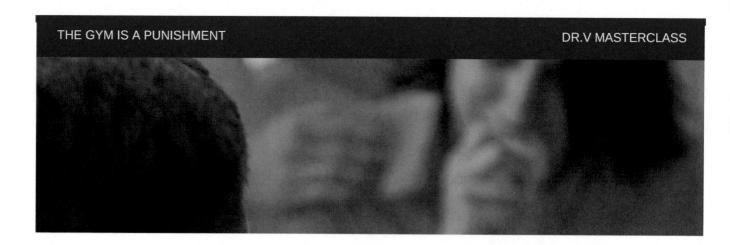

IS YOUR HEAD STRAIGHT?

THE GYM WILL NOT FIX THE SOURCE OF YOUR OBESITY.

Your obesity did not come out of thin air. It is a penalty of years of bad habits, choices, and belief systems. These things all have a source. And until you deal with it, the thing that triggered your spiral into obesity is still there--a hidden landmine waiting to be triggered.

So before you think of the gym, you need to think of the source and deal with it. Where did these bad habits and beliefs come from?

Did you get so busy that fast food was easier than home cooking? Did marriage problems lead to comfort eating? Did a childhood trauma contribute to the lethargy of depression? Did a relative instill a belief like 'food makes everything better' or that a clean plate somehow honored the starving children in Africa?

Knowing why you eat- or do any other unhealthy habit - is the key to controlling triggers and old behaviors. Instead of the gym, look into more productive things like self-help, counseling, coping techniques, stress management, fixing current day problems, and anything else interfering with your thoughts and moods.

Your head is on straight when you have a handle on the problems. The gym is only a temporary distraction at best, not a solution.

> Patients tell me all the time that they use the gym to work out their stress. This belief is UNHEALTHY. Why? Because when they get home, the source of their stress is still there. Gym for stress is a *distraction*, not a solution!

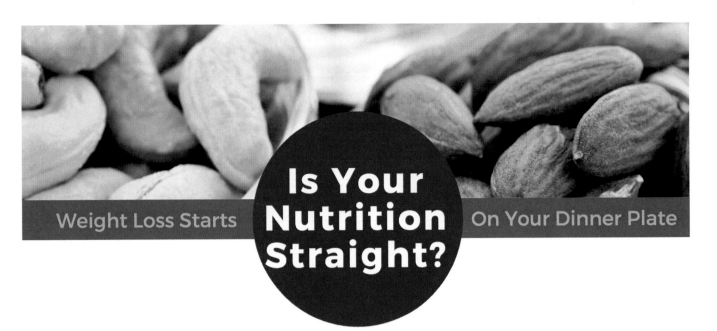

Is Your Nutrition Straight?

Weight Loss Starts On Your Dinner Plate

You can not exercise off a bad diet. Bad food choices will immediately counteract anything you try to do regarding weight loss. And a bad diet will not give you the nutrition you need to use the gym for other goals, like gaining strength.

Before you even think about the gym, get your eating habits in order. Get used to hydrating with water instead of sweet drinks. Stop snacking altogether. Make drinking a green smoothie for necessary nutrition second nature. Learn how to get most of your minerals and proteins from plant-based foods.

A few tips to get started:

Take the money you would have spent at the gym and use it on fresh ingredients, a good smoothie blender, and other equipment you need at home to train yourself to a better diet.

Box up all the bad snacks, sodas, and pre-processed foods still in the house and get rid of them today. Throw them out. Don't hold onto them for treats. Don't leave them there for a 'quick fix.' Don't tempt yourself with a bad habit.

Use the hour you would have spent in the gym researching healthy recipes, learning alternatives to your old cravings, and other useful things to get your food-habits back in order. If you are stuck on where to start, my book *Eating Healthy on a Budget* will tell you how to make small practical changes right away.

Real Talk With Dr V

Some patients try to tell me that because they are exercising, any weight gain is "muscle". Not so. Factors vary, but in general, to gain one pound of muscle in a week you have to consume 14 extra grams of protein, 500 extra calories **beyond what you will burn off** and follow a rigorous training routine that keeps it from becoming fat [3]. **Rapid weight regain is NOT muscle gain.**

THE GYM IS A PUNISHMENT DR.V MASTERCLASS

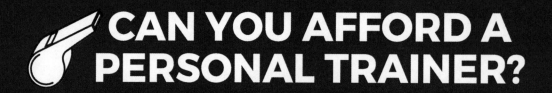

CAN YOU AFFORD A PERSONAL TRAINER?

A personal trainer is the single most important piece of gym equipment you will need. If you can't afford one, or a higher membership with a personal trainer included- You are not ready for the gym. Period. No arguments or exceptions.

 They help you set realistic goals unique to you.

 They keep you from injuring yourself with instruction and realistic focus on your needs.

 They help you work on mobility and stability, as well as weak core muscles.

If you don't hire a physical trainer, you are almost guaranteed to injure yourself. You'll try to do what you think you can do, or what you see the trimmer and fitter people are doing. You'll pull muscles, overstress your body, and possibly injure yourself on unfamiliar equipment. If you can't afford a personal trainer- it is not worth it. Even IF you don't injure yourself, you will have wasted a lot of time and effort, when there was a faster and better way to get to your goals.

Ideally, you should look into physical therapy first. It is an atmosphere custom made to help you build up stability and mobility. Then if you want to work on heart health, stamina, or other specific goals, save up for a personal trainer to work on targetted goals later- once you also have your head straight and your nutrition straight!

HEALTHY WAYS TO GO AFTER GOALS

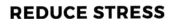

REDUCE STRESS

Deal with the source(s) of stress.
Meditation
Find a hobby away from food.
Positive and supportive people
Counseling

WEIGHT LOSS

No Snacks
Drink 80-100 oz of Water
Avoid "sports" drinks
Make healthier food choices

FIT BODY

Patience- It takes years to sculpt
Take pride in loose skin- it means
you are losing the weight.
Physical Therapy to build up core

GET HEALTHY

Better food choices
Better hydration
Better sleep habits
Follow doctor's orders
Guided Physical Therapy

The Gym is not the place to advance your weight loss goals.

You won't feel good.

It will make you hungry

It will sabotage your new lifestyle

And it won't help you
LOSE WEIGHT

So don't punish yourself. Focus on your goals and come back to the idea of the gym when you have everything else straight first.

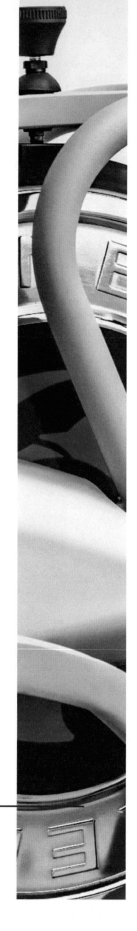

Am I Ready?

WRITE DOWN ANYTHING YOU NEED TO WORK ON. USE THE NEXT PAGE TO FOCUS ON THESE THINGS INSTEAD OF THE GYM.

IS MY HEAD ON STRAIGHT? Y / N

IS MY NUTRITION STRAIGHT? Y / N

CAN I AFFORD A PERSONAL TRAINER? Y / N

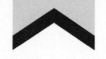

GETTING ON TRACK
MONTHLY PLANNER

MONTHLY FOCUS

- [ ] ....
- [ ] ....
- [ ] ....
- [ ] ....
- [ ] ....

DATES TO REMEMBER

....

....

....

....

....

NOTES

GOALS

- [ ] ....
- [ ] ....
- [ ] ....
- [ ] ....
- [ ] ....
- [ ] ....
- [ ] ....
- [ ] ....
- [ ] ....
- [ ] ....
- [ ] ....

[1] Ainsworth BE, Haskell WL, Herrmann SD, et al. 2011 Compendium of Physical Activities. Medicine & Science in Sports & Exercise. 2011;43(8):1575-1581. doi:10.1249/mss.0b013e31821ece12

[2]Judy A. Driskell, Ira Wolinsky. 1999. Energy-Yielding Macronutrients and Energy Metabolism in Sports Nutrition: Nutrition in Exercise & Sport.

[3] Lally, P., van Jaarsveld, C. H. M., Potts, H. W. W., & Wardle, J. (2010). How are habits formed: Modelling habit formation in the real world. European Journal of Social Psychology, 40, 998-1009

MASTERCLASS 5

Conquer Hunger Forever

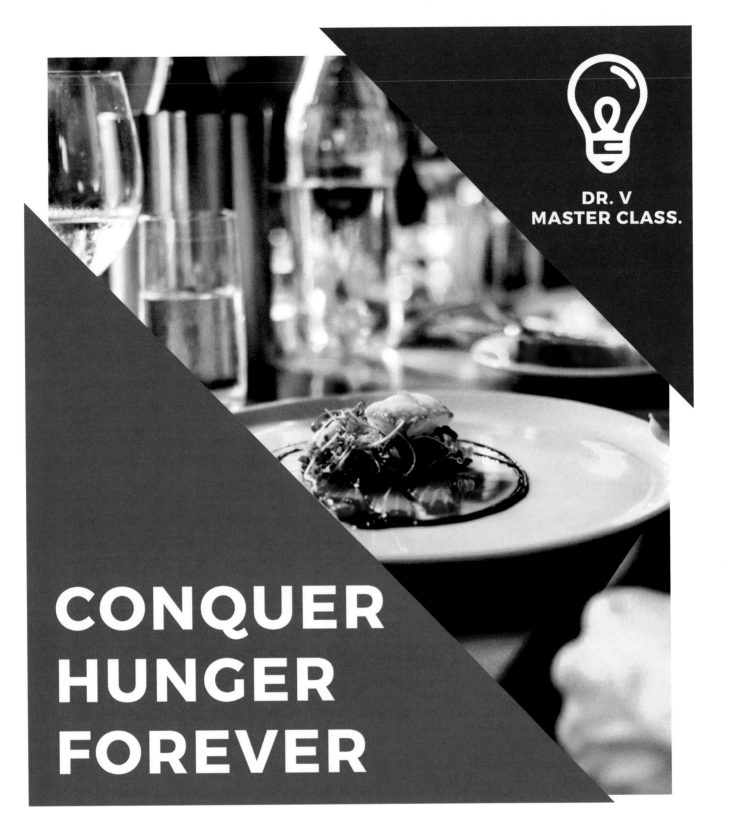

CONQUER HUNGER FOREVER

DR. V
MASTER CLASS.

PRESENTED BY

Dr. Duc Vuong

WHAT IS HUNGER?

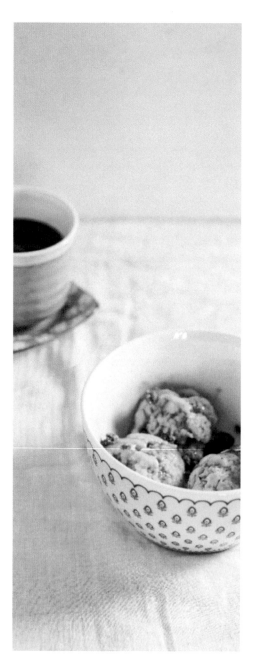

Hunger is defined in the Oxford dictionary in two distinct ways. In the first, it is categorized as "a feeling of discomfort or weakness caused by a lack of food, **coupled with a desire to eat."**

Of course, this first definition looks great on paper. However, what about when we have eaten enough food to be full but still feel hungry? In this instance, the second definition becomes relevant:

"A strong desire or craving."

In short, hunger is your body's way of requesting nourishment and fuel for its everyday needs. However, it is that growling in your gut, the watering of your mouth, that nagging thought in the back of your head saying "I need this food *now!*" that is the actual source of frustration for many people.

I will show you how to control this once and for all!

We are taught *hunger is bad*. It is an undesirable condition that means we lack something. Our entire culture revolves around fast, easily accessed foods that are designed to make us feel 'full' for a little while.

The problem? We did not evolve with easy access to empty calories! During prehistoric times, we were usually without food and rarely had enough to eat to be full. In other words:

It's Natural to be Hungry.
It's Unnatural to be Full.

WHERE DOES HUNGER COME FROM?

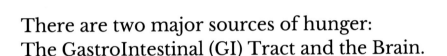

There are two major sources of hunger:
The GastroIntestinal (GI) Tract and the Brain.

The GI tract is a huge producer of hormones that affect various body functions. The Brain, in turn, responds to these signals with tits own set of chemicals, which leads to the emotions, rationalizations, and hunger responses that drive us to eat.

In 2005 science discovered what was dubbed as Ghrelin, otherwise known as the Hunger Hormone. Its job was to travel to the brain and trigger a hunger response sequence. Even today, studies are showing a connection between this hormone and food cravings [1].

Initially, we believed we found the 'magic button' to obesity. If we could suppress this hormone, we could control hunger. However, even with weight loss surgery, medications, and proper eating habits: *The hunger always eventually returns*. WHY?

That is because...

Your Body is Super Redundant!

As of 2017, we have discovered 20-25 hormones in the body that affects hunger and satiety. Why so many? Because our bodies are designed to survive. If something happened to one hand, you have another. If one kidney fails, you have a second to take the load. The same goes for your hunger system.

Why so many? **Because eating used to be tedious. We** had to organize a hunt. We traveled for supplies. Broke down the kill. Cleaned up after so other predators wouldn't get it. Without a system to drive us to eat, it would have all the appeal of doing any other chore three times a day, 365 days a year for the rest of our lives.

But this tedious task is necessary to keep us ALIVE. So, the body has multiple backup systems. Eventually, these systems bypass any breaks in the system (weight loss surgery, pills, or diets) and hormones resume their trek to the brain. This means...

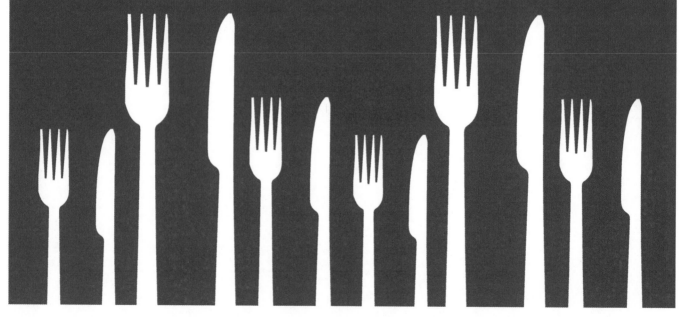

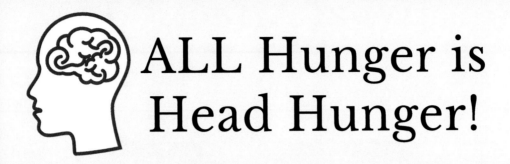 ALL Hunger is Head Hunger!

While hormones travel to and from the brain, they are only a reporting system. *It is the brain that spurs you into action.* We do not crave food until we *think* about wanting it.

Skeptical? Think about a time you got so engrossed in something that nothing else registered. Maybe it was a book, or an art project. Maybe it was a game you couldn't put down. Or a very engaging conversation. Or you were stressed over an upcoming test. Then it ended, and then the hunger flared up.

The hormones were there. The empty belly was present. Your blood sugar and automatic body functions did their natural responses--but you did not notice any of the hunger alarms while this activity captivated your attention, i.e. brain.

ALL hunger is Head Hunger because food is not a factor until you are conscious of it. Likewise, you will hold off acting on that hunger until you *choose* to stop and find something to eat.

All hunger has a thought process to it, whether we notice those thoughts or not. It all comes down to things that lead us to act on hunger.

What Affects My Hunger?

Here are just a few of the various factors that affect hunger and eating patterns

CULTURE

What society at large accepts

- Common Foods are heavy in fats, starches, carbs and sodium.
- Convenience food culture.
- Easy Access to cheap foods

HABITS

Things you do at specific times, places, and events

- Chips with a movie
- A dessert after dinner
- The morning coffee stop on way to work
- The afternoon soda
- The pizza party after a game

SOCIAL

How you treat food with others

- Eating unhealthy foods to fit in.
- Extra snacking while socializing.
- The one relative who keeps piling your plate because you are 'too skinny.'

HEALTH

How well nourished and efficient the body is

- Cravings sometimes indicate a nutrition gap where body is low on a key nutrient
- Blood sugar and insulin levels can affect cravings [2]

EMOTIONS

- Eating out of loneliness or boredom
- ."Comfort" foods
- Sweets and other snacks boost "feel good" dopamine levels [3].

STRESS

- Acute stress hinders appetite, while chronic stress increases cravings for fats and sugars [1].

EXTERNAL FACTORS

Things outside yourself, such as the smell of apple pie or a tv commercial.

INTERNAL FACTORS

Your personal influences, such as your memories, culture, emotional state, and habits.

TIPS TO CONTROL HUNGER

- Hydrate and Wait. Sometimes the body confuses low-level dehydration with hunger. Drink 8 oz (half a bottle) of water and wait 15 minutes to see if the craving ebbs.

- Check for Physical Signs. If your stomach isn't growling and you have no warning signs of hunger, reassess what might be triggering the event.

- Do Something Else. If it it is boredom, the hunger will fade when the mind is occupied.

- Light Exercise. Activity through the day is shown to positively affect mood, energy and appetite [4].

- Replace Food based rewards with healthier alternatives, like self-praise or time for a favorite activity.

- Smaller, Slower Portions. Savor food, and give your body time to register fullness.

- Change Meetups. Instead of meeting at a pizza shop, meet at a park, a healthy smoothie shop, or other place where unhealthy temptations are not so handy.

- Get Household on Board. Make home a no junk-food zone. Establish better family habits.

- Don't Freak Out! If you slip, just accept it as a slip and continue your health goals. Focus on long term results.

HOW TO PRACTICE MINDFUL EATING

Mindfulness is the act of staying aware and present. With all the distractions of the world, it is a challenge to come to a full stop and think of what we are putting into our bodies. Here are a few simple ways to get started.

1. Ask Why You Want to Eat. Are you Actually hungry? Or Bored? Stressed? Rushed? Is it hunger or do you feel obligated to order something when you go out to socialize? Differentiating between a need to eat and a want to eat is a huge first step to avoiding unneeded calories.

2. Question Your Food Choices. Do you crave the chip? Or do you crave the saltiness? The crunch? Is there something similar with better nutrition to it?

3. No Multitasking. Put the phone away. Turn off the tv. Stop, and sit down to only eat. Distracted eating leads to you consuming way more than you would have

4. Cook Your Own Food From Scratch. When you cook your food, you have to pay more attention to the ingredients going into your body. If you stick to healthy, nutrient-rich ingredients, this will also make things like salads your new "fast food."

5. Eat Slowly and Savor. Chew each bite 20 times and take notice of the texture and flavor. It will help you register when you are full, and you will feel full and satisfied with less. [5].

6. Be Aware of Portions. Don't eat straight out of a bag or pre-packaged container. Take out the appropriate amount and put it on a plate so you can *see* how much you are eating. Likewise, go with smaller plates or serving sizes when you eat out.

You can also find more tips and simple exercises in my book *Meditate to Lose Weight*, available on Amazon.

Parting Words:

We are taught to see hunger as "bad."

But Hunger is Natural,
Fullness is Unnatural.

Question: Who never feels hungry?
Answer: Dead People

Your New Mantra

"I'm Hungry.
That makes me happy.
Because it means I am alive!"

MY HUNGER TRACKER

Instructions: Print out and use this sheet to track the internal and external things that make you crave food. The goal is to target and control your food triggers.

EXTERNAL

-
-
-
-
-
-
-
-

INTERNAL

-
-
-
-
-
-
-
-

MEALS

TODAY I DEALT WITH HUNGER BY:

OTHER NOTES

CONQUER HUNGER FOREVER

DR. V MASTERCLASS

[1] Chao, A. M., Jastreboff, A. M., White, M. A., Grilo, C. M. and Sinha, R. (2017), Stress, cortisol, and other appetite-related hormones: Prospective prediction of 6-month changes in food cravings and weight. Obesity, 25: 713-720. doi:10.1002/oby.21790

[2] Martina Guthoff, Yuko Grichisch, Carlos Canova, Otto Tschritter, Ralf Veit, Manfred Hallschmid, Hans-Ulrich Häring, Hubert Preissl, Anita M. Hennige, Andreas Fritsche; Insulin Modulates Food-Related Activity in the Central Nervous System, The Journal of Clinical Endocrinology & Metabolism, Volume 95, Issue 2, 1 February 2010, Pages 748–755, https://doi.org/10.1210/jc.2009-1677

[3] Caroline Davis, Natalie J. Loxton, Robert D. Levitan, Allan S. Kaplan, Jacqueline C. Carter, James L. Kennedy Corrigendum to "'Food addiction' and its association with a dopaminergic multilocus genetic profile" *Physiology & Behavior*, Volume 149, 1 October 2015

[4] Audrey Bergouignan-Kristina Legget-Nathan Jong-Elizabeth Kealey-Janet Nikolovski-Jack Groppel-Chris Jordan-Raphaela O'Day-James Hill-Daniel Bessesen - Effect Of Frequent Interruptions Of Prolonged Sitting on Self-perceived Levels Of Energy, Mood, Food Cravings and Cognitive Function. https://ijbnpa.biomedcentral.com/articles/10.1186/s12966-016-0437-z

[5] Angelopoulos T, Kokkinos A, Liaskos C, et al The effect of slow spaced eating on hunger and satiety in overweight and obese patients with type 2 diabetes mellitus BMJ Open Diabetes Research and Care 2014;2:e000013. doi: 10.1136/bmjdrc-2013-000013

MASTERCLASS 6
Breaking Bad Food Habits

WE REFUSE TO TAKE THE STEERING WHEEL

Avoiding the Responsibility of Change

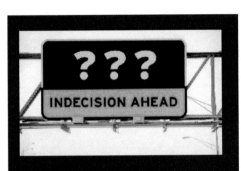

"I'LL 'TRY' TO CUT DOWN ON MY SNACKING."

"I NEED SOMEONE TO TELL ME HOW FIRST."

"OH WELL, NO BIG DEAL THIS ONE TIME."

"I WANT TO, BUT I'LL MISS..."

"I'M TOO ADDICTED TO FOOD TO MAKE THIS WORK."

Changing eating habits requires a full lifestyle commitment. You *actively* no longer fall back on your favorite comfort foods. The way you treat holidays is different. The way you interact with friends about food is different. The activities you pursue no longer come with snacks. Even the way you prepare for meals is different.

And you are fully aware of every change, and 100% of it is your responsibility.

Accepting personal responsibility for all these changes is tough. While it means we reap the benefits and avoid the path our ruts were taking us, it also means we are responsible for our failures and frustrations as well.

It's easier to avoid the change. At least it is a devil we know. We can blame other things for our weight gain: our food addictions, our doctors, our circumstances. And all the things we like and are comfortable with stay the same.

HOWEVER-
NOTHING CHANGES.

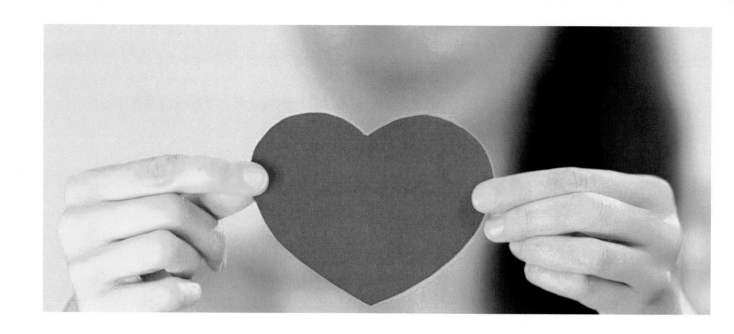

Why Did You Have Weight Loss Surgery?

You went thought WLS for one reason: **You wanted your life to change**. You wanted to be healthier. You wanted to feel better. You wanted the weight bearing aches and pains to stop. You wanted to do things like walk and climb stairs without effort. You wanted to lose the weight that is holding you back.

But to change your life, you have to change the things that caused your troubles in the first place: **The foods you eat and why you eat them.**

If you want to change your life, you can *not* be complacent in your eating habits. You **can't** keep doing the one thing that made you obese in the first place.

"No one wants to go through the therapy, testing, and surgery involved in WLS just to go back to their old lives"
-- Dr. V

Taking Back the Steering Wheel

To succeed in your new life, there is one thing you MUST do. It is the cornerstone that will make or break your goals and efforts.

You have to CHOOSE to engage in healthier eating habits. Every meal. Every scenario. Every day.

Food habits are like an addiction. You will feel discomfort and frustration in the beginning stages of withdrawal. You will even feel strong cravings and buyer's remorse for the choice to live a more mindful eating lifestyle.

Your success in resisting and overcoming setbacks will depend on how strong your conviction is.

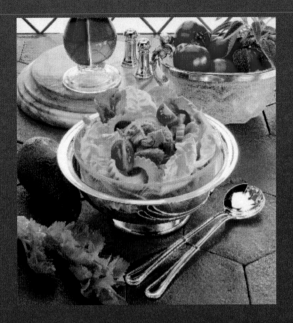

"Food addicts have to make the active choice to avoid their old eating habits" – Dr. V

You have to do more than just *stop*.

You have to actively make the decisions to eat healthier. Every day for the rest of your life. Once you put your hands back on the steering wheel, you have to keep them there. You can not rely on your ruts to pull you mindlessly along like you did in the past.

Once you fully and completely invest into actively changing your life, you will be ready to start into healthier habits. Let's go over a few essentials.

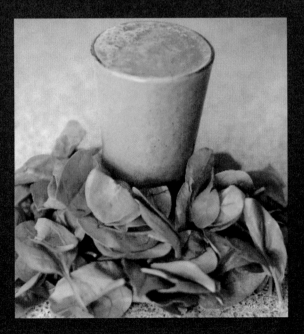

BREAKING BAD FOOD HABITS

DR. V MASTERCLASS

Tips To Change Eating Habits

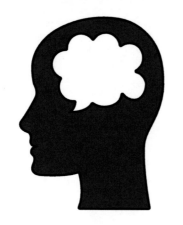

Get to the Root of Your Habits. Your food choices didn't happen in a vacuum. Dealing with the source of each unhealthy food habit will make it easier to get healthy. Therapy and mindfulness will be essential as you build a new foundation.

Deal With Bad Habits that Affect Eating. For example, poor sleep habits are linked to higher cravings and snacking [3][4].

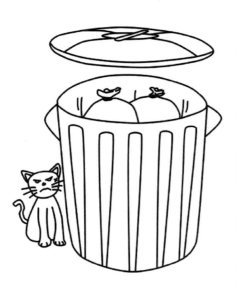

GET RID OF TEMPTATIONS

Throw out all unhealthy food. Don't think about waste. Don't save it for a rainy day.

Change meeting places with friends to areas you won't be surrounded by food and sweet beverages.

BUY AND PREPARE YOUR OWN INGREDIENTS

Green Smoothies: A green smoothie for breakfast will give you all the calories and nutrition you need to get through the morning.

Salads: We're talking more than a pile of iceburg lettuce. Learn the various and delicious recipes that make a salad a filling meal.

Make Your Own Meals: It is the only way to control how fresh and healthy your food is. Cooking basic fresh foods like baked fish, roasted peppers, and Quinoa take no cooking skill whatsoever.

Learn how to store and freeze extra portions for future meals.

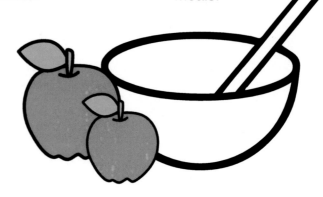

Find more tips, resources, and recipes in my books on Amazon.

KEEPING YOUR HANDS ON THE WHEEL

How to Stay Mindful and Accountable

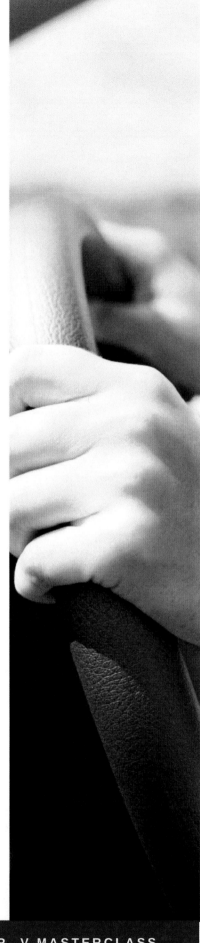

Question Your Hunger. Hunger is normal, but a specific mind-trigger made it noticeable. Are you physically hungry or just going along with a habit? Drink a glass of water instead of snacking.

Practice Mindful Eating. Slow down and savor your food. Chew everything 20 times.

Learn to Meditate. Slowing down and letting your mind regroup will reduce both fatigue and bad food choices.

Keep a Gratitude Journal and a Food Journal to track your progress over time.

Gravitate to people who will support and encourage your new eating habits. If certain people try to criticise or sabotage your work, resolve to spend less time with them, or avoid them altogether.

Be proud of your accomplishments. Post before and after shots and milestones on your social media page. Don't listen to complainers. You're doing it for you and no one else.

Find a motivational partner or team to share triumphs and setbacks with.

Stick with your therapy and follow-up appointments. Be honest with your healthcare professionals and support teams. Love them when they tell you if you are moving in the wrong direction. If they don't say anything, then they are complicit in your bad health.

Be Patient, but no excuses. It takes a bare minimum of 66 days to change a habit, often longer [5]. If you mess up, don't try to validate or minimalize it. Calmly think over what happened, how you can do better next time, and keep moving forward.

FINAL THOUGHTS
IT'S YOUR LIFE, CHOOSE TO GIVE IT YOUR BEST

Put your decision to break your bad eating habits down in writing.

Don't just think about getting healthier. Don't wait for a magic solution. Don't hedge your bets with 'trying.' Resolve to make the choices that will lead you to better health.

You are the only person at your steering wheel. It's up to you to grab hold and guide yourself to the changes you desire most.

Don't Talk.
DO!

NEW HABITS JOURNAL

"We are what we repeatedly do. Excellence, then, is not an act, but a habit."
--Aristotle

GOALS FOR TODAY

_____
_____
_____
_____
_____

TODAY I ATE:

_____
_____
_____

TODAY I AM MEETING MY HEALTH GOALS BY

_____
_____
_____
_____
_____

TODAY I AM GRATEFUL FOR

_____
_____
_____
_____
_____
_____
_____
_____
_____

I NEED TO WORK ON

_____
_____
_____
_____
_____

[1] Kate, P. E., Deshmukh, G. P., Datir, R. P., & Rao, J. K. (2017). Good Mood Foods. J Nutr Health Food Eng, 7(4), 00246.

[2] Wurtman, J., & Wurtman, R. (2018). The Trajectory from Mood to Obesity. Current obesity reports, 7(1), 1-5.

[3] K. Spiegel, E. Tasali, P. Penev, and E. Van Cauter, "Brief communication: sleep curtailment in healthy young men is associated with decreased leptin levels, elevated ghrelin levels, and increased hunger and appetite," Annals of Internal Medicine, vol. 141, no. 11, pp. 846–850, 2004.

[4] Nedeltcheva, A V et al. "Sleep Curtailment Is Accompanied by Increased Intake of Calories From Snacks." American Journal of Clinical Nutrition 89.1 (2008): 126–

[5] Lally, P., van Jaarsveld, C. H. M., Potts, H. W. W., & Wardle, J. (2010). How are habits formed: Modelling habit formation in the real world. European Journal of Social Psychology, 40, 998-1009 133.

MASTERCLASS 7
Conquering Criticism

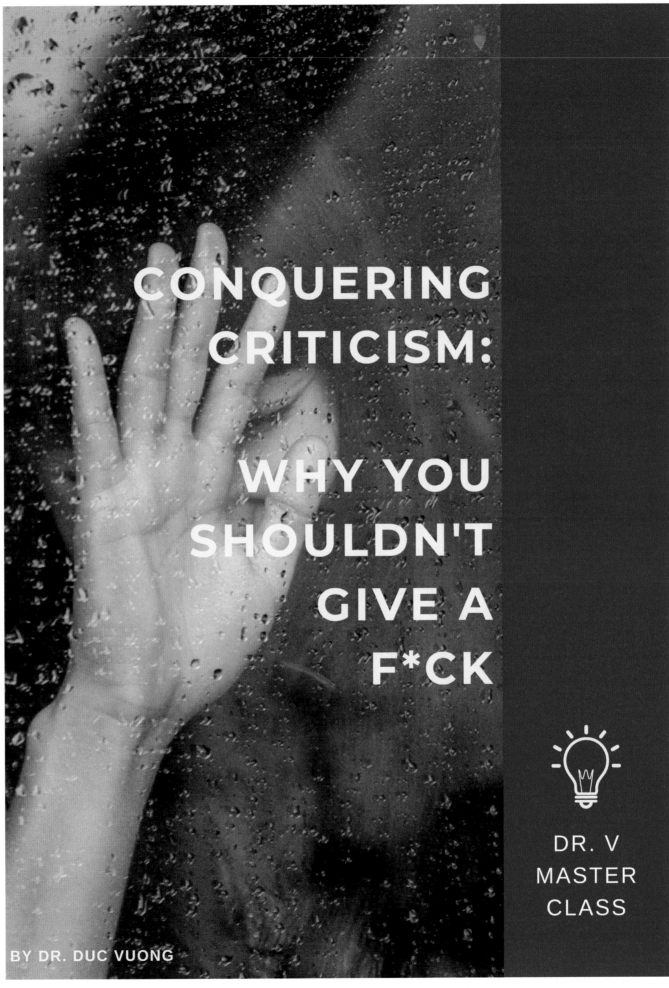

CONQUERING CRITICISM:

WHY YOU SHOULDN'T GIVE A F*CK

DR. V
MASTER
CLASS

BY DR. DUC VUONG

DOES IT FEEL LIKE ALL EYES ARE ON YOU?

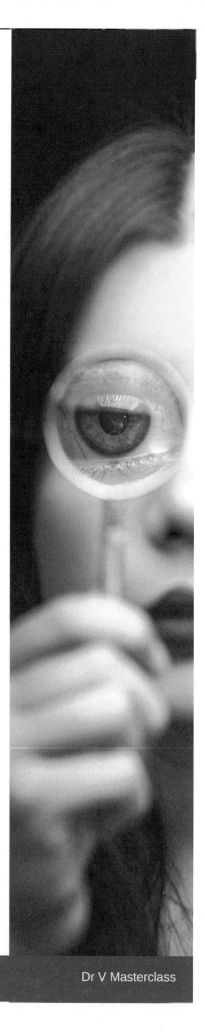

Criticism is an inevitable part of our life journey. There will always be someone that has something to say--whether it is about our taste in music, our beliefs, or our habits.

It only becomes a problem when we place *value* on what others might think.

If you are afraid to be criticized by others, it *will* affect your daily happiness.

Have you ever held back due to what people might say? Did you ever skip a promotion because you were worried how co-workers would treat you afterwards? Drop a huge dream because others thought it was unrealistic? Do you avoid drinking your green smoothie in front of others because you didn't want to be labeled a "health freak"? Do you avoid publicly recording your triumphs because you don't want to look like a braggart?

We are going to address some surprising facts about criticism, including the simple truths that will set you free from its *illusionary* power over your life.

In a few short pages, you will have a simple and immediate path toward big success and true freedom to live your life.

WHY WE OBSESS OVER WHAT OTHERS THINK

- **We Are Social Creatures**. We want to feel important to others. This need is so strong that if we value the person's opinion, *social pain can be as painful as physical pain* [1]. This is a big issue in our modern culture, where we even value the opinions of strangers on the internet.

- **We Let Our Minds Wander**. Keeping focused takes mindfulness and active training on positive and proactive things. If we do not focus and obsess on the right things, then we will obsess on average and trivial things that catch our attention, such as the latest work gossip or family drama.

- **Negativity Dominates**. We are surrounded by negative news, gossip, weather-related disasters, and other emotional downers. We have a strong desire to always be "in the know" with the latest news, so we will seem interesting to others. But if you do not work at staying positive and self-motivated, your mind and attitudes absorb that negativity and affect your behavior. Then finding no positives in yourself, you seek validation from external sources, such as Facebook.

- **Deflecting Responsibility**. When we focus on the fear of criticism from others, we are *making excuses and trying to place the blame of failure outside ourselves*. However, you and only you are responsible for your choices.

Self-Criticism

Be careful how you are talking to yourself because you are listening.
-- **Lisa M. Hayes**

It's bad enough that we let what others think stop us from our dreams; but what's worse is that we do it to ourselves. Self-Criticism is a major obstacle that can tear down your efforts and even keep you from getting started in the first place.

In my practice, 69% of my patients dropped out before they had their surgery. And many of the remaining 31% would say discouraging things about themselves like "I am a slow loser" or "I don't have the willpower to control my cravings."

How you talk to yourself will determine how you act. It affects how much energy you put into a goal. It affects how you view your progress. It affects if you will quit when things get challenging.

Your thoughts determine your success or failure more than any other factor. Not even biology or natural talent can withstand the limits we speak on ourselves.

There are two truths you must embrace in order to free yourself from the power of negative thoughts and opinions.

THE TWO MIND-BLOWING TRUTHS

NO ONE IS THINKING ABOUT YOU BECAUSE THEY ARE TOO BUSY THINKING ABOUT THEMSELVES

These people that you are so worried about are busy with their own lives. They don't have TIME to obsess over your life. They are not keeping themselves up at night over you. Even if they are, they won't be 5-minutes from now.

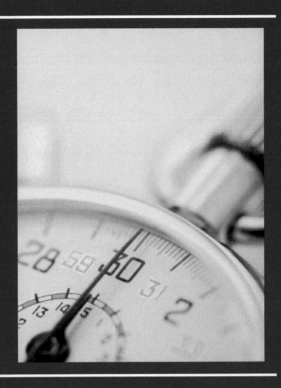

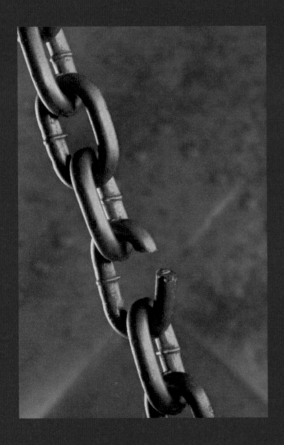

IF THAT'S TRUE, THEN DO WHAT THE F*CK YOU WANT! STOP USING FEAR OF CRITICISM AS AN EXCUSE TO KEEP YOU FROM YOUR TRUE HAPPINESS.

You do not have time to obsess over their opinions. You have *only* one life to live, and you are the *only one* responsible for it.

Since no one is actually thinking about your life, you have the freedom to do with it what you truly desire.

YOU HAVE PERMISSION TO BE AWESOME

Since no one is losing any sleep thinking about what you do, you might as well be awesome in the process. At the end of the day, you are only accountable to yourself.

So dream big, make lofty goals, and plan out your path to success.

Record and celebrate your achievements without flinching at the eye rolls and snubs of average people trapped in their own negativity.

Chase that promotion or pursue the studies that lead to your dream job. Write that book you talked about for years. Find new recipes for your healthy eating goals. Travel to some region you've only seen in magazines or on Instagram.

You have one life. No do-overs or take backs. Make sure to live the rest of it in a way where you have no regrets when you reach the end of your life.

Now some of you are probably thinking "Dr. V, that's easy to say. But I don't have the money or the talent to do *THAT*."

Here is a secret for you: Success has nothing to do with wealth OR talent. All successful people, without fail, share one trait...

SUCCESSFUL PEOPLE ARE OBSESSIVE

- Sachin Tendulkar is the only person to score 30,000 runs in international cricket [2]. Imagine how well you could do *anything* after repeating it 30,000 times.

- Thomas Edison filed over 1000 patents in his lifetime.

- The famous French fashion designer Coco Chanel stated "Fashion is not something that exists in dresses only. Fashion is in the sky, in the street, fashion has to do with ideas, the way we live, what is happening [3]."

No matter where you turn, successful people all have one thing in common: They invest a huge sum of time, energy and thought into the ONE THING they eventually become known for. They didn't succeed with half-hearted efforts. They didn't make excuses or wait for approval. They obsessed over their goals until success was the only possible outcome.

This is exactly what you need to do to achieve all your dreams and overcome criticism. And to do that you need to...

RETRAIN YOUR BRAIN

- **Write Your Goals**. Put them on record and track your progress. It is scientifically proven that writing down goals has an effect on your health and your success rate [4]. There is a worksheet at the end to help you get started.

- **Be Obsessive About You**. Show your goals the same energy and passion people give their favorite tv show. Use that driving energy that ensures they never miss an episode on getting your daily green smoothie. Talk about your goals and milestones with that same zeal as they do their favorite character. Be as heedless to eye-rolls and blank stares as they are when revealing your latest developments toward your goal. Read personal development books. Watch YouTube videos on personal growth. Go to conferences.

- **Set alarms** and calendar alerts, and name them with your goals and affirmations. Review your goals and practice your meditations or gratitude journals during times of criticism to refocus.

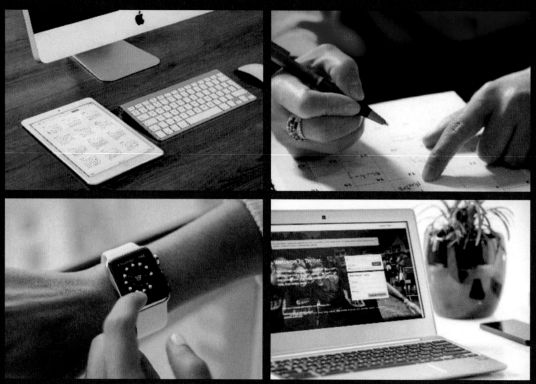

You do not NEED to worry about what other people are thinking about you. They are busy obsessing over their own lives.

You do not NEED to fill your head with doubts and self-criticism. Self-loathing does not get you anywhere and will NEVER fix ANY of your problems.

You NEED to *retrain your brain* and start obsessing over yourself and *your* goals. No matter what you decide to do, make sure to be awesome at it.

Whatever You Do, Do it BIG! Success will Follow.

Dreaming Big

BECAUSE I AM FREE TO BE AWESOME, I WANT TO...

_____

_____

_____

_____

_____

TO ACCOMPLISH THIS I NEED TO

☐

☐

☐

☐

NOTES

_____

_____

_____

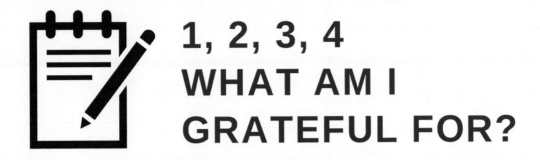

1, 2, 3, 4
WHAT AM I
GRATEFUL FOR?

**SPEND THE NEXT 1 TO 2 MINUTES WRITING ALL THE
POSITIVES IN YOUR LIFE THAT YOU CAN THINK OF.**

[1] Cook, G., & Cook, G. (2018). Why We Are Wired to Connect. Scientific American. Retrieved 10 July 2018, from https://www.scientificamerican.com/article/why-we-are-wired-to-connect/

[2]Sachin Tendulkar Biography. (2018). Biography Online. Retrieved 10 July 2018, from https://www.biographyonline.net/sport/cricketers/sachin-tendulkar.html

[3] Coco Chanel Biography. (2018). Biography Online. Retrieved 10 July 2018, from https://www.biographyonline.net/artists/coco-chanel.html

[4]King, L. A. (2001). The health benefits of writing about life goals. Personality and Social Psychology Bulletin, 27(7), 798-807.

MASTERCLASS 8
Dealing with Loose Skin

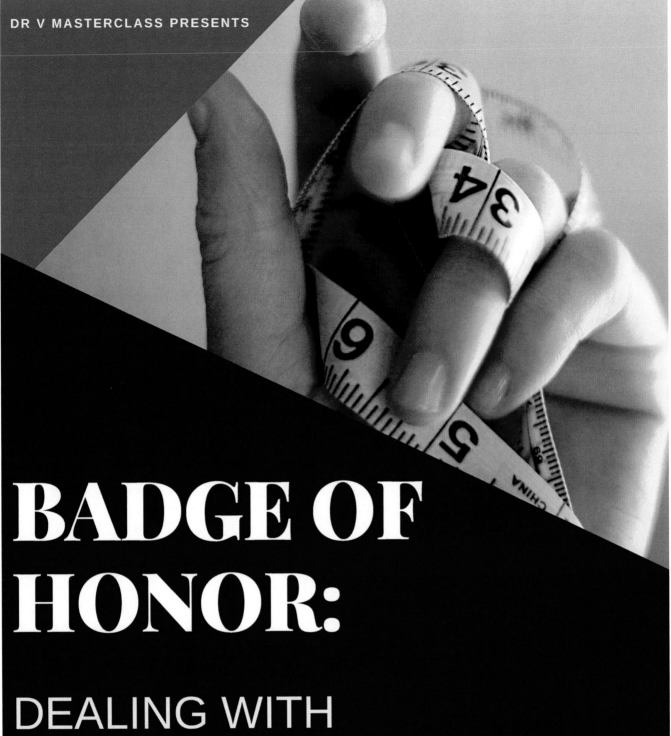

BADGE OF HONOR:

DEALING WITH LOOSE SKIN AND PLASTIC SURGERY

BY DR DUC VUONG

LOOSE SKIN IS A REALITY OF WEIGHT LOSS

Loose skin is also something to be proud of. It is living proof that you have conquered your habits and lost the weight that has plagued you. Today my message to you is that **loose skin is a badge of honor**. Wear it proudly.

In this report, I'll go through some surgical and non-surgical ways to manage it:

- The limits of nonsurgical methods
- Conditions where insurance might pay for plastic surgery
- The mental side of plastic surgery
- Ways to build up the money you need in as little as two years.

LOOSE SKIN IS

A BADGE OF HONOR

1%
OF PEOPLE WHO QUALIFY FOR WEIGHT LOSS SURGERY ACTUALLY HAVE SURGERY

15%
GET THE SURGERY AND FAIL TO LOSE ANY WEIGHT [1]

58%
SUCCEED AT SIGNIFICANT WEIGHT LOSS LONG TERM [1]

It is almost guaranteed that if you lose weight, you are going to have loose skin. And that is a good thing! Look at these stats- over 99% of your peers who qualify for weight loss surgery at the same time as you *will not get the loose skin because they won't follow through*. They will self-sabotage, ignore their current health situation, and fail to make the changes needed to create a healthy lifestyle.

Bat-wings, turkey necks, loose thighs and other loose skin is proof positive that you beat the odds. It is a mark of success. A reminder of how far you've come.

That means **loose skin is your new goal**! It's the badge of honor you wear to show your commitment to this journey. And it is a badge you can trade for battle scars with plastic surgery if you so choose.

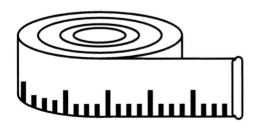

"BEFORE YOU WORRY ABOUT LOOSE SKIN, YOU'VE GOTTA GET THERE FIRST!"--Dr. V

- **Get Your Priorities Straight**. Your physical and mental health is more important than what you'll look like with a skin apron. Don't hold back or self-sabotage. Your heart, arteries, and back do not care what your skin looks like; They care about how they are straining under the extra fat that they are not *designed* to maintain. Your Health-Related Quality of Life (HRQL) is far more important than saggy skin [2].

- **Make Your Plans Now**. If you think you will want to do surgery or procedures when you've lost the weight, start saving today. You can't lose. You will either have money saved for skin removal surgery or a lump of savings for other life goals. If you find yourself not bothered by your loose skin, you can use the money to take a trip to an exotic place, go back to school, or other life-enriching events.

- **Learn to Not Give a F&@K! About What Other People Think**. People are gonna talk...but luckily they don't have time to think about you for more than five minutes. They are busy dealing with their own stuff. Don't let their five minutes of opinion ruin your progress.

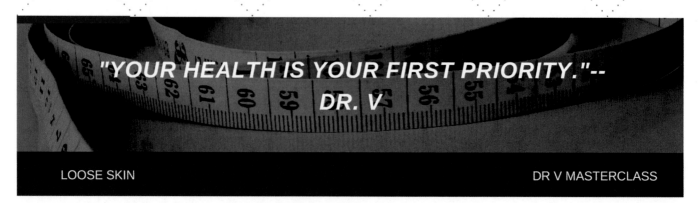

"YOUR HEALTH IS YOUR FIRST PRIORITY."--DR. V

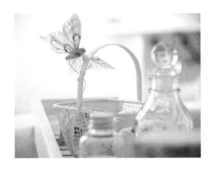

CREAMS

Skin firming creams and serums can help with mild loose skin, wrinkles and stretch marks left to improve the overall look. But they will NOT eliminate skin aprons.

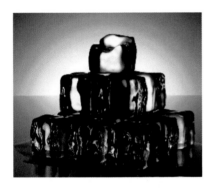

COOL SCULPTING

Cryolipolysis, or 'cool sculpting' freezes and kills fat cells while promoting collagen growth. It is best for body contouring and treating small localized areas, such as fixing a pouch left behind from surgery [3].

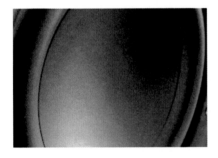

ULTRASOUND WAVES

Studies show that Ultrasound therapy is effective in increasing collagen and skin elasticity, and tightens mildly loose skin [4].

Keep in mind that these methods do not remove your loose skin. They help with trouble spots that need contouring and shaping. These are also strictly cosmetic, so your insurance will not cover it.

There is only one way to deal with the large areas of loose skin...

PLASTIC SURGERY IS THE ONLY WAY TO REMOVE LOOSE SKIN

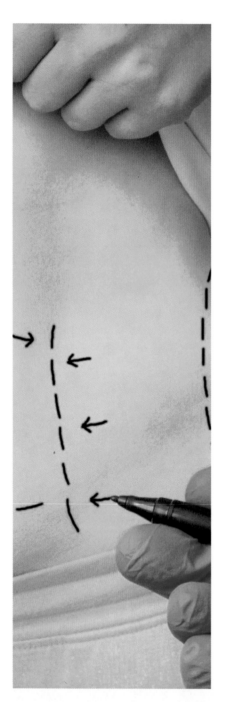

Many patients assume they can exercise away loose skin. **This is false**.

Think of your loose skin as an overstretched piece of clothing: no matter how much you move and exercise, your clothing will not get smaller.

Exercise is good for toning your muscles, strengthening your heart and lungs, and maintaining your weight. It will improve your overall health...but not sagging skin.

A plastic surgeon is the ONLY SOLUTION. Just like a tailor, they take that overstretched clothing, cut away the excess, and sew it together for a better fit. They are experts in dealing with weakened abdominal muscles, sagging breasts, and undesirable fat folds that come from massive weight loss.

BUT there is one vital point you must always keep in mind...

YOU WON'T LOOK LIKE THE PICTURE IN YOUR HEAD

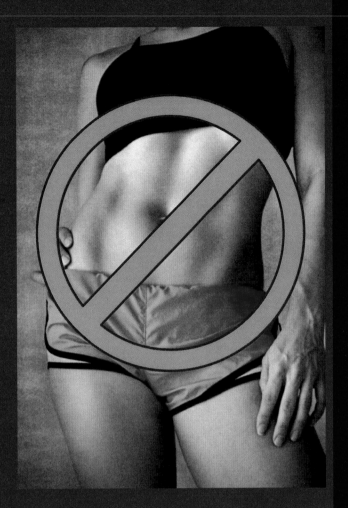

Plastic surgery is not going to give you that perfect figure. Multiple plastic surgeries won't give you that Hollywood superfit bikini model body **you see in your head.**

Plastic surgery is about cutting away the excess skin and getting sewn back together. You will be more comfortable, but *there will be scars*. Large and noticeable scars (that you can sometimes hide) to replace the apron and bat wings.

Plastic surgery is a trade-off. Skin for scars. Less noticeable but still annoying fat dimples. Drainage tubes as you heal. A painful recovery. It's not the glamorous little nips and tucks portrayed on television.

This does not mean the surgery is a waste of time. But you do need to make sure you are doing it for the right reasons:

- You WILL fit into clothing better.
- You WILL be more comfortable.
- You WILL endure fewer issues like back pain and rashes.
- You WILL NOT magically erase away the body image issues.

WILL MY INSURANCE
PAY FOR PLASTIC SURGERY?

1. Some states have more leeway than others. In New Mexico, we are fortunate to have a few surgeons that accept insurance.

2. Insurance has to Allow for Health-Related Surgery. Not all insurances are created equal, and many are only for emergency care, preventative treatments, etc.

3. Have to Explain That It is Not Cosmetic. Plastic surgery is not usually covered because it is considered a cosmetic procedure. In order for insurance to pay, you have to prove that you are doing it for health-related reasons like back pain, rashes, fungal infections, etc.

4. Documentation. Whenever your loose skin is causing you a health-related issue, you have to document it. Don't ignore symptoms. Go to the doctor to put rashes and pain on record. Make sure you and doctor take pictures and put the conditions on record. It will greatly increase your chances of having the surgery covered for medical reasons.

Keep in mind that these will not guarantee that your insurance will cover the plastic surgery. These are factors that must be present to increase your odds of approval.

So what if insurance does not cover your surgery? Or requires you to pay a substantial co-pay?

DO THE MATH: PAYING FOR YOUR PLASTIC SURGERY

GOAL	2 YEARS	2.7 YEARS	5 YEARS
$10,000	$13.69/DAY	$10/DAY	$5.48/DAY
$20,000	$27.38/DAY	$20/DAY	$10.96/DAY

The price of plastic surgery varies widely based on your location, the specialist, and how much area you are working on. But in ballpark figures, you should be prepared to spend between $10,000 and $20,000 for surgery.

That may seem like a lot of money, but look at how much we spend on a new car. Anywhere from $15,000 to over $50,000 - and that is not even touching the luxury car models. And that is for something we use a few hours a day at most, often far less. Your surgery is an investment in your body, something you use 24 hours a day, 7 days a week, until the day you die.

Look at the five-year column above. Most people spend more than that a day just for specialty coffees. If you can spend $5-$15 a day on nonessential expenses- you can save it too.

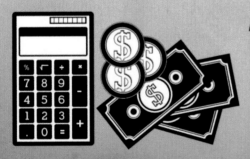

Let's go over a few of the hundreds of ways you can save money for your surgery without hurting your budget, starting with my favorite and most effective one:

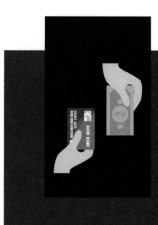

DR. V'S DEBIT CARD STRATEGY

Every time you use your debit card, check to see if there is a cash back option. Withdraw as much as you are allowed without harming your budget for the month. Take that money home and immediately hide it away. Then forget it. Don't talk about it. Don't tell people it exists. Don't ever take it from its spot for any financial reason. Just accumulate it until you are ready for surgery.

You won't miss it, I promise you. When you think of all the impulse buys that usually landed in your cart before your eating habits changed, you have a lot more leeway for this trick than you think.

I am living proof. I used this trick to save up when I was broke. I could always withdraw $5 to put away for my goals. When things got better, I took out more. I never missed it month to month, and I got closer to my goal every time.

There are two tricks to this: You must not dwell on it. You have to pull the money, stash it, and forget it. And you must not under any circumstance take it out for anything but your goal.

And in TWO SHORT YEARS you will have either money for your surgery or a huge lump sum to change some other part of your life. Win-win!

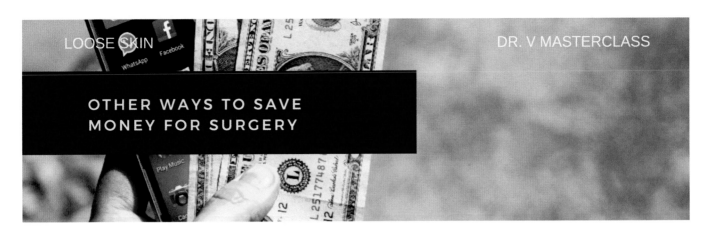

OTHER WAYS TO SAVE MONEY FOR SURGERY

- Immediately place any income outside your normal monthly budget in your savings for surgery: tax returns, season bonuses, rebates, that $20 someone repaid two years later...

- Cut redundant fees- do you really need cable, Netflix **and** Hulu in one month? Or an internet fee **and** a phone data plan? Put the cost of any discontinued subscriptions straight into your savings every month.

- Don't pay a "Convenience Fee"- put the money you would have paid for delivery, no-commercial plans, and rush shipping memberships into your surgery savings instead.

- Acorns, Stash, and other sites help you save by investing a set amount of funds for you on a regular basis. In addition, some have features like rounding up purchases to the nearest dollar and investing the difference. Because it is automated, you don't need to think about investing these funds.

- Health Goal Reward apps let you record your progress via a phone or fitness tracker and reward points for healthy tasks you achieve. Find some that offer PayPal or monetary rewards, then place any reward income into your surgery savings.

- Find ways to make a side income: Freelancing, house-cleaning, sitting, selling on e-bay, etc. Put all income from this side venture away for surgery. When you meet your goal, you have an established side hustle to continue saving for the next big thing.

Someday vs. Day One

Don't get caught in the trap 'Someday I will...' The perfect conditions you are waiting for to start 'someday' will never come. To succeed, you need to start acting. Instead say, "Today is Day One!"--Dr. V

Loose skin is a Badge of Honor.

Physical proof that you have changed your life for the better.

If needed, you can manage it.

You can even get rid of it through plastic surgery for your health or as a secondary goal.
Plus you can develop a skill to earn extra income.

BUT NEVER BE *ASHAMED* OF YOUR LOOSE SKIN!!!

[1] Snyder, B., Nguyen, A., Scarbourough, T., Yu, S., & Wilson, E. (2009). Comparison of those who succeed in losing significant excessive weight after bariatric surgery and those who fail. Surgical endoscopy, 23(10), 2302.

[2]Jia, H., & Lubetkin, E. I. (2005). The impact of obesity on health-related quality-of-life in the general adult US population. Journal of public health, 27(2), 156-164.

[3] Ingargiola, M. J., Motakef, S., Chung, M. T., Vasconez, H. C., & Sasaki, G. H. (2015). Cryolipolysis for fat reduction and body contouring: safety and efficacy of current treatment paradigms. Plastic and reconstructive surgery, 135(6), 1581.

[4] Minkis, K., & Alam, M. (2014). Ultrasound Skin Tightening. Dermatologic Clinics, 32(1), 71–77. doi:10.1016/j.det.2013.09.001

MASTERCLASS 9

Emergency Money

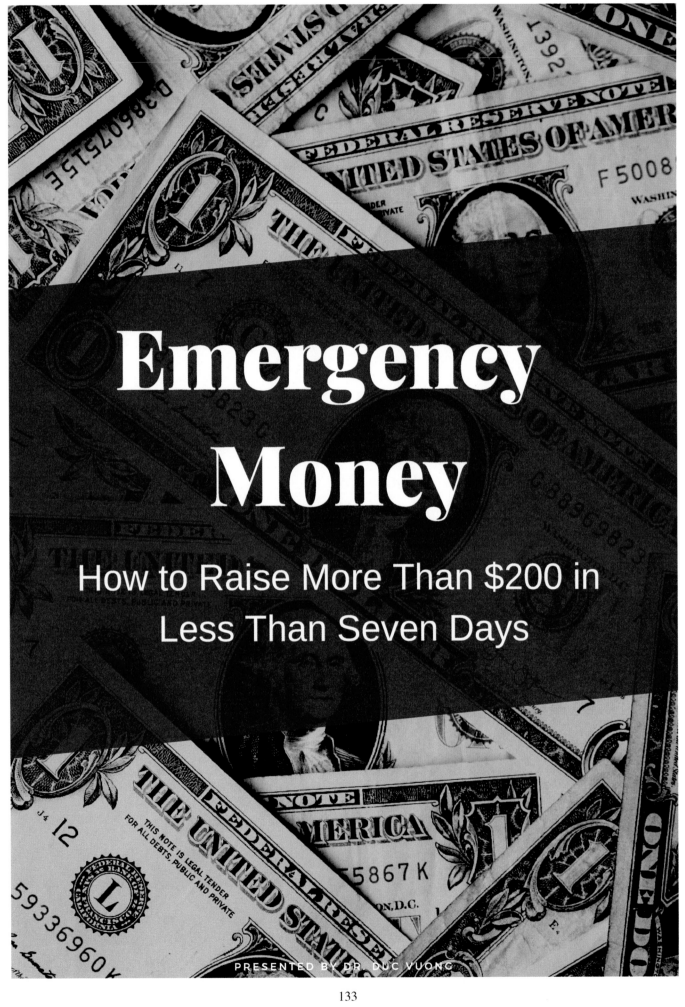

Emergency Money

How to Raise More Than $200 in Less Than Seven Days

PRESENTED BY DR. DUC VUONG

EXPENSES BIGGER THAN YOUR BUDGET?

It happens to the best of us. Some months there are too many expenses and too little paycheck. It could be from a higher than expected utility bill, medical issues, a broken down appliance, kid's school costs, or any number of obstacles and inconveniences life throws at us.

Still, when you are looking at a couple hundred dollars more in costs than your income can handle, the hurdle to take care of all your responsibilities can feel daunting.

We're going to go over a few ways you can draw out an extra $200 in a week to cover those unexpected issues AND ways to help reduce the chances of getting stuck again.

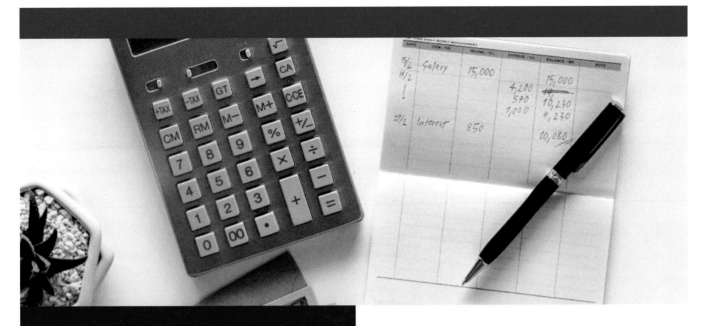

Before you try to fix the problem, you need to understand why the problem happened. This goes beyond the immediate issue. Why was there not a fund set aside for these situations in the first place?

You have to take a long, hard look at all your income and expenses, including your bills, subscriptions, convenience fees, and even the pocket money you hand your kids for the store.

Getting a hard, honest look at your finances will make solving the issue easier, as you'll have to face the impulse buys, unused memberships, redundant costs, and more.

Questions to Ask:

- What am I paying for that I am not using? (gym memberships, video streaming, audio book service, etc)
- What am I paying for twice? (Cable AND Netflix, Cell AND a Landline, etc).
- What "plans" can be suspended or cancelled until things improve?
- What expenses have a cheaper alternative?
- What am I spending on unplanned purchases?

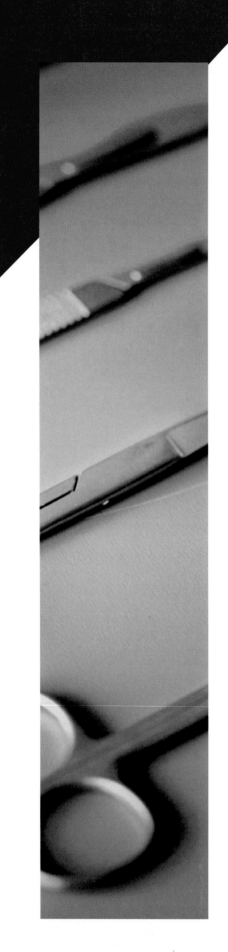

CUT COSTS

Once you've taken a hard look at your expenses, it's time to cut out all the waste. After that, you'll be able to:

- Allocate any immediate savings to the current crisis, dropping your actual needed income.
- Free up part of your income for an emergency savings account. You'll be more prepared for future financial crunches.

Promptly cut out any unnecessary expenses--unused memberships, unread magazines/newspapers, the lesser used of your video streaming services, 2-day delivery memberships, etc.

Next go through all of your utilities and call the customer loyalty department of each to see if you can downsize or renegotiate your terms with them. If your contract is up, also look at their competitors to see if you can get better service at a better deal somewhere else.

Learn the tips and tricks to avoid high costs. For example, your electric company may charge a lower fee if you avoid the laundry and vacuuming until a certain time of day, and solar curtains help regulate the amount of heat you fight during the summer.

You can stack store sales, store coupons, and manufacturer's coupons on a single item. And most stores have a designated discount area for things they need to liquidate.

Whatever you can save from your immediate expenses, put immediately into the gap in your finances.

Enjoy Life On Less

Does this mean you have to cut out all the fun stuff? Not at all! You should stick to free entertainment options until you get past the immediate crisis -- but overall you just need to find cost efficient ways to enjoy life. For example:

--Libraries are more than book clubs. Some have free workshops, Crafting and experimenting classes for kids, cultural demonstrations, and even language and yoga classes.

--A picnic at the park, pool, or hiking trail can make for a day of fresh air, exercise, and memories. Don't forget to take plenty of water!

--Some restaurants let kids eat free on certain week nights. You can check for a fun (*healthy*) family night on sites like mykidseatfree.com

--State fair in town or child wants to see the zoo for their birthday? Check discount sites like Groupon and Stubhub for discounted admission costs on *memory-making* events.

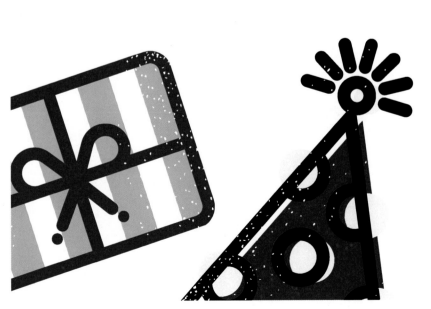
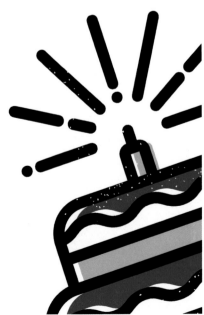

Clutter to Cash

The fastest way to make extra money outside employment is by selling off stuff you don't need.

A yard sale, secondhand store, and sites like Bookoo and eBay are places you can exchange your stuff for the funds you need this week.

There are several upsides. You clear out space. You have a few less things collecting dust around the house. And you have cash in hand to put toward your financial crisis immediately with no strings attached.

If you need to sell fast, expect many items to sell for way less than you paid for them.

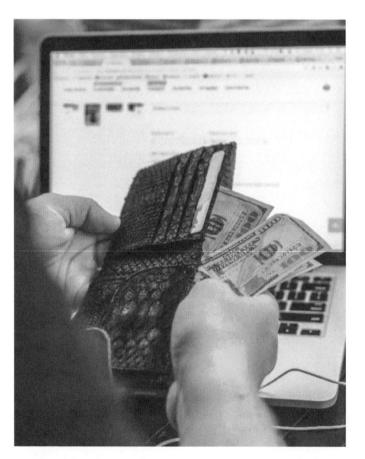

- Furniture and fairly current electronics will sell the fastest at the highest price.
- Collectibles like comics or mint condition cards will sell best to specialized shops or buyer areas vs a general sale.
- Sell old baby clothes and gently used kids toys.
- You can sell high end clothing through consignment shops or sites like Threadup.
- Sell gift cards at a discounted price.
- Antiques and "vintage" items sell fairly quickly if you advertise to the right people or antique resale shops.
- You can sell old dvds,cds and other electronics in lots or on sites like Decluttr.com

There is a market for just about everything you own, though some will sell faster than others.

RENT YOUR STUFF

There are sites that will act as a middle man to help you rent your room, spare storage, or even your carport, lawnmower, or xbox.

Renting your space and stuff is useful in that it remains yours once the time period is up. It also means you can make a repeated income off the same items later.

Make sure you are in compliance with any leases, city regulations and zoning laws before signing up for this option.

A FEW EXAMPLES ARE:

- Extra Bedrooms - AirBnb
- Yard equipment, games, and other high end items- Zilock.com
- Parking Space- Justpark.com
- Clothing- Loanables.com
- Travel gear- Ayoopa.com
- Spare Car- Turo.com

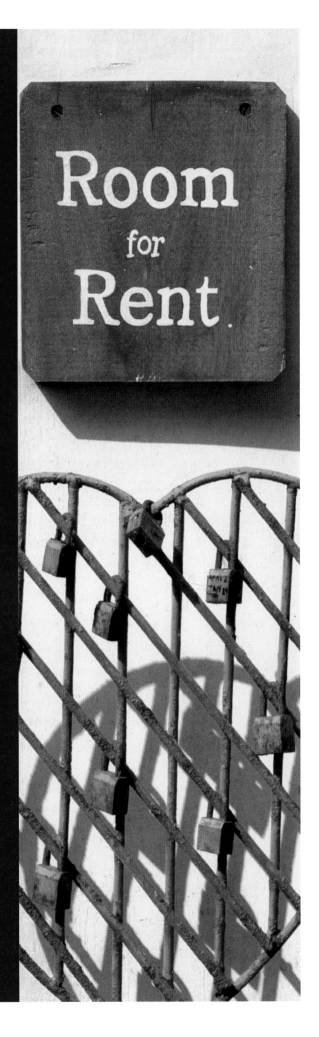

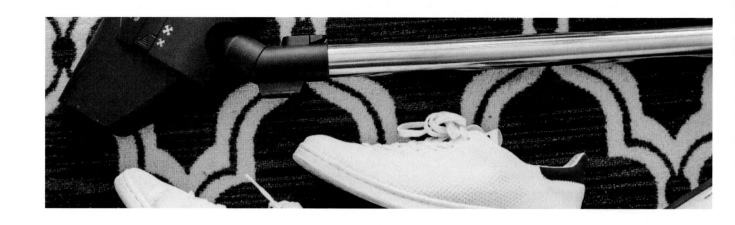

FILL A NEED

In today's hectic race, there are always people willing to pay for one less thing to worry about, or more quality care for their loved ones. And you do not need to resort to flyers and newspaper ads.

If you have the extra time, you can make quick money with the traditional babysitting, cleaning, and life skills like basic handiwork. Here are a few sites you can set up your profile and begin to find clients quickly:

Pet-sitting: Rover.com
Dog walking: Fetch.com
Babysitting or eldercare: Care.com
Grocery Shopping: Instacart.com
Housecleaning or Handiwork: Taskrabbit.com
Driving/Taxi: Uber and Lyft
Delivery: Postmates, Ubereats, Amazon Flex

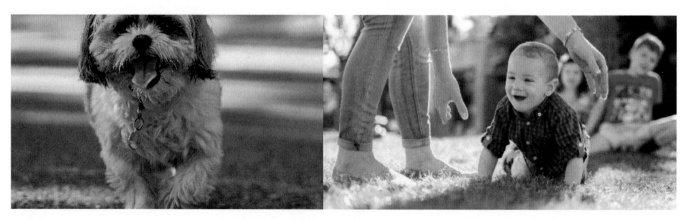

BE A VOICE

We live in a very connected world, and businesses are willing to pay for that human touch for their brands.

Needle.com: Advocate for your favorite brands by talking to shoppers.

Carvertise: Advertise brands on your vehicle

Erlibird: Test Aps

Focusgroup.com: Tell companies what you think

GoTranscript: Listen to and write audio files into documents.

Usertesting.com: Test out websites as a normal viewer and report how user friendly it is (or is not).

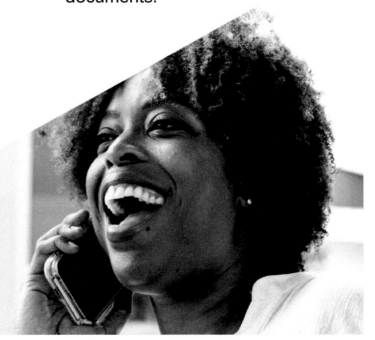

Community Aid

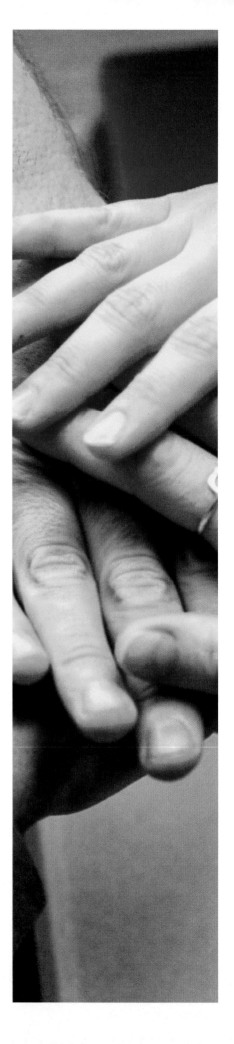

Many communities have some sort of assistance available to them. Some larger churches and community centers have a benevolence program where they help people in a temporary crisis with one utility bill, groceries, or even rent. If you need extra funds due to a temporary situation out of your control, reaching out can often be a helpful means to handle it.

The terms are often strict, with a long cool down before you can ask for aid again. But if they agree to assist you with any vital bill, it will reduce your financial burden by that much more.

Whatever expense they can help with, reallocate that budget to the current issue.

Not keen on charity? Donate back to their programs with volunteer time, resources, or funding once your situation has improved.

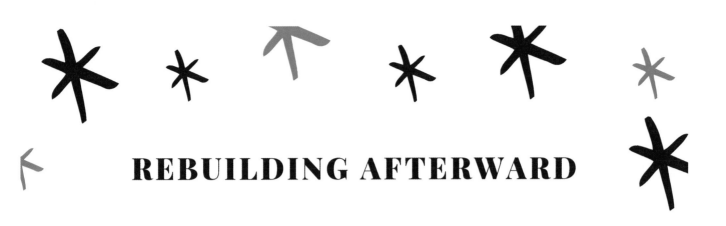

REBUILDING AFTERWARD

HOW TO BUILD UP FUNDS FOR GOALS AND FUTURE EMERGENCIES

- **Dr V's Debit Card Trick**: Every time you use your debit card, take out as much as you can afford to without harming your budget. IMMEDIATELY put it away out of sight. Don't touch this money until the exact reason you are putting it away for comes up.
- **Auto-stash**. Sign up for an app that automatically withdraws a specific amount of funds for you on a set schedule. These sites often have investment options in micro-stocks and bonds as well!
- Keep doing any jobs, rentals, etc you picked up to get through this crisis. Put ALL funds from it into an account separate from your budget account, this money is for emergencies and *meaningful* expenses/goals that enrich life in some way, like a leadership camp, class, etc.
- Put any extra windfalls (refund checks, rebates, etc) into a jar or separate account from your budget.
- **DISCIPLINE!** Do not give into the temptation to spend your money on needless things or extra conveniences. You may have to sell them for way less than you paid in the next financial emergency. Keep your eye on your budget and make sure each dollar counts.

CONCLUSION

You can take control of your money emergencies.

1 Find the problem—including the impulse buys and excessive spending.

2 Cut back any unnecessary costs and put any budget savings toward the problem.

3 Monetize your extra stuff and your skills. Seek out any aid available.

4 Start building an emergency account for future issues. Put any surplus budget into this account immediately so that it is not spent until you consciously choose to.

Life Happens.

You can keep control of your finances whenever a curve ball hits.

Keep calm. Give the issue a hard, honest look. Go through your opportunities.

When you get past the crisis, make sure to build up so you are more prepared for the next one.

PLANNING SHEET

I Need to increase my
available funds an extra
$_____ by __ / __ / __

WHAT CAN I CUT FROM MY EXISTING
BUDGET? (CABLE, ALCOHOL, FEES)

_____

_____

_____

_____

WHAT CAN I SELL? (UNUSED GIFTS,
FURNITURE, TRINKETS)

_____

_____

_____

_____

WHAT SKILLS CAN I OFFER? (HOUSE
CLEANING, BABYSITTING, SALES)

_____

_____

_____

_____

MASTERCLASS 10

Mind Games

Mind Games:
How to Control Fear of
Failure After WLS

By Dr. Duc Vuong

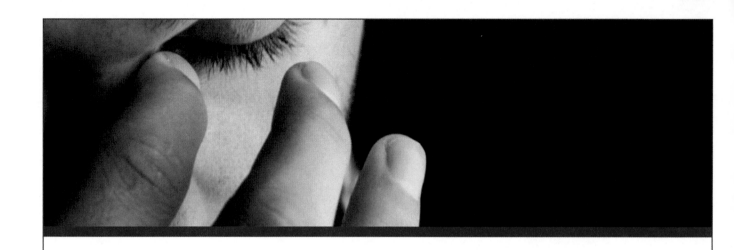

INTRODUCTION

Our thoughts are powerful. They can build us up or tear us down. They can move us forward or hold us back. Motivate us to succeed or sabotage us into failure.

Negative thoughts and wrong beliefs do not stop after surgery. In fact, they get worse, especially once unfamiliarity sets in. It's not all roses and rainbows, Dorothy.

The months and years after surgery are all about change. Your body is changing. Your relationships are shifting. Your diet and eating habits have undergone a huge overhaul.

However- the surgery only affected parts of your body. The messed up thoughts that react to fear and change are still haunting your head. But your old way of handling fear and stress--EATING--is now gone.

This means that if you are not careful, you will try to deal with your new reality with old thoughts that created the obesity mess in the first place. Getting past these problems is going to take work.

In this report, I will discuss the three most common mind games that interfere with weight loss after surgery. **You will learn techniques to beat those mind games.** By the time we are done, you will have the tools necessary to control the mind games that hold you back.

THE TWO CORE EMOTIONS

There are two and only two emotions, LOVE or FEAR. Every other emotion is related to these two. Even powerful emotions like hate and jealousy are rooted in fear.

When you experience healthy levels of love and fear, you are able to take reasonable actions and think through consequences in an equally reasonable manner.

However, the thoughts and fears that led to your obesity, whether they were traumatic or negligent, are not under your control...yet.

Work towards feeling enough love for yourself so you can escape the mind games and focus instead on the changes that will maintain your healthier life style.

LOVE

Love motivates us into action. Love for the people around us. Love for our lives. Love for ourselves.

When we love something, we try harder to fulfill goals related to it. It is the most powerful counter-measure against fear-driven thoughts and behaviors.

FEAR

In ancient times, fear kept us alive. It was a mechanism to keep us from doing things that could cause us harm.

However, fear also keeps us from doing things that are good for us as well. Fear tries to demotivate us from taking unfamiliar actions. But it's the unfamiliar that leads to growth.

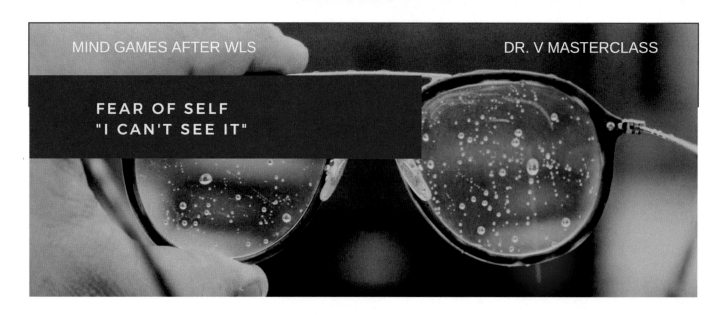

**FEAR OF SELF
"I CAN'T SEE IT"**

There is a very high rate of mood disorders like **chronic anxiety** and **depression** in the population of people that seek out bariatric surgery[1]. And even after surgery, many people experience such negative self-perception that they engage in self-harm [2]. This is why is it extremely important not to ignore the mental exercises related to your surgery: Meditation, Journalling, Therapy, etc.

Before you go in for surgery, it is important to do the mind work. Surgery will not fix the root of the problems that caused your obesity in the first place. It also will not magically fix your self-perception or other mental baggage.

One of the most common things I hear during the weight loss process is the phrase "I can't see it..."

Mostly, this comes from the people who have been obese all their lives and have never seen themselves as anything but "that fat person." Others are the ones that thought a single therapy visit right before surgery would be enough to fix any issues. Also, others that can't see any positive progress do some work, but they do not do it with the focus and learning to make it effective.

In the end, they all share one thing: They hide from the issues that affect their self-image. It takes work to change the way you think about yourself. You can not finish the recovery process unless you can face yourself with all your flaws, fears, shortcomings and insecurities. **You have to love yourself enough to make the changes necessary to overcome them.**

Real Talk With Dr. V

If you aren't seeing the changes, you aren't doing the mental work!
To battle negative self-image you have to learn to love and acknowledge yourself.
Half-hearted attempts or simply 'knowing' what you should do won't cut it.

Fear Your Relationships Will Change

All of your relationships will change. That is a given.

This can be a terrifying realization. Our relationships are **comfortable habits**. Change means that things will no longer be comfortable and predictable. You have to learn how to deal with these new realities all over again. Even a positive change can feel a little nerve-wracking. **You must learn to be comfortable with being uncomfortable.** Here are a few changes you can expect to deal with:

Marriage/Family

You'll find some of your relationships will improve. You'll notice some people are more supportive and praise your efforts.

Likewise, you will notice that some relationships are not working out. They will distance themselves ("Is that ALL you're going to eat?") or outright try to sabotage your efforts ("You've been so good, this one time won't hurt...")

Work

As your looks and confidence improve, you'll start experiencing positive changes in your workplace, like more focus and energy. You may see a raise, offers for training, and possibly a promotion.

You may also encounter unsupportive co-workers that harbor some fear, envy or insecurity in your change. Or you may come to the sudden realization that you can do better and look for another workplace.

Friends/ Social Circles

Birds of a Feather Flock Together.

You are the average of the five people you most associate with. As you lose weight and establish a healthier lifestyle, you will find yourself distancing from some of the people you associate with. Others may even drift off on their own. You'll find yourself spending more time with the people who support or live the same healthy lifestyle.

Two Unexpected Relationships That Will Change

YOUR RELATIONSHIP WITH FOOD

We do not always think about our food when we think about relationships. However, it is one of the most important ones that will change.

Food is engraved into your concept of self. Dishes you make that people love. Your old favorites. The way you seek comfort or celebrate. All these things and more are part of your relationship with food.

The problem is that it was a very unhealthy relationship, and this unhealthy relationship caused your obesity. Your surgery gives you the opportunity to totally redefine your relationship with food for the better.

The hardest part will be getting past the head hunger. Each lost habit creates a vacuum, and nature hates a vacuum. That's when the mind games start. You will eat your portion and be physically full. You will have received adequate nutrition, but you might suddenly feel an overwhelming frustration--**you will want to eat more**. You will HATE the fact that you CAN'T have one more bite. You may even feel buyer's remorse, i.e. miss your old comfort foods, miss snacking, miss sweets.

As you develop a better relationship with your food, these struggles will grow less intense. And this will ultimately affect...

YOUR RELATIONSHIP WITH YOURSELF

If you lose 100 pounds or more, which is the average weight of a cheerleader, you will have lost a whole person (and by then many habits that put those 100+ pounds on you). **You are literally a different person from the one that went in for surgery**.

The mind games start when you try to behave like that new person. You think differently. You see the world differently. You interact differently. You need to put in the work to treat yourself differently too, otherwise the mind games and insecurities **will lead to self-sabotage**.

YOUR #1 FEAR: WEIGHT REGAIN

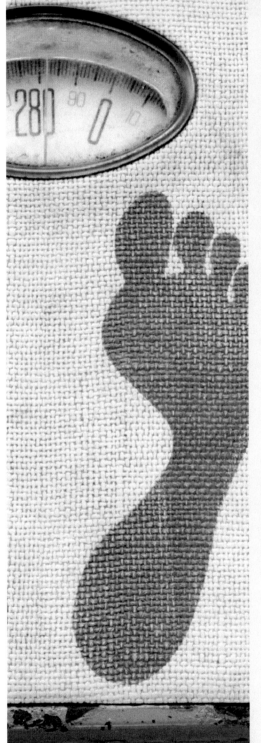

The fear of regaining weight is common post-surgery and stems from a deeper fear[1][3]. You lost control once to head hunger, and you paid the price.

In a healthy mind, the fear is easy to control. The only thing that can make you gain or lose weight is the food you put into your body. If you stick to your diet, work closely with your medical team, and use your surgery correctly, you will become healthier and not regain the weight.

But fear is not logical, especially when it is linked to a much deeper fear that we might not realize or acknowledge. The result: even though people know the right way to keep the weight off, they react to a deeper fear linked to their weight.

Self-monitoring and developing a love for oneself are the key countermeasures. Ideally, you work at things like journaling and meditation the rest of your life to keep this fear in a healthy and manageable range.

There are two types of fear that drive the fear of weight regain. Each one has its own behavior pattern...

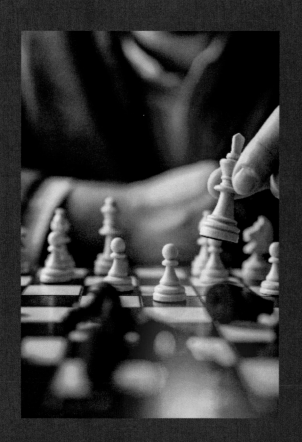

1. OBSESSIVE FEAR

Causes worry, concern, obnoxious behavior, and OCD-like attention to every carb and calorie.

The excessive attempts to control food shows a fear of the lack of control.

"If I slip, I will fail."

2. PASSIVE FEAR

In contrast, with passive fear you are so afraid of failure that you are paralyzed by it. You know the choices you make will undo your weight loss efforts. You know you need to make changes. But you don't try or put in the effort.

"I don't know" and "It doesn't matter" are common reactions to this type.

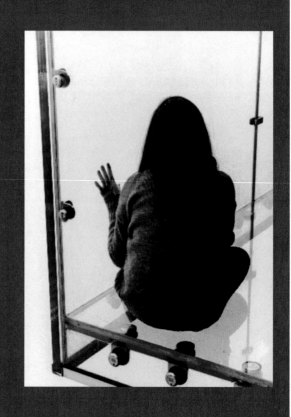

Tips to Battle Mind Games

Learn and practice proper journaling. This is an essential skill to see the progress you make. You must journal to give yourself documented proof of progress to combat the mind games and insecurities [3].

Learn basic meditation and practice it daily. Meditation is not magic. It is a simple practice of removing distractions and letting your brain focus solely on you.

Deal with your relationships. If you have a bad marriage, get counseling or a divorce lawyer. If a toxic friend is trying to get you to eat bad food, set your boundaries or distance yourself from them.

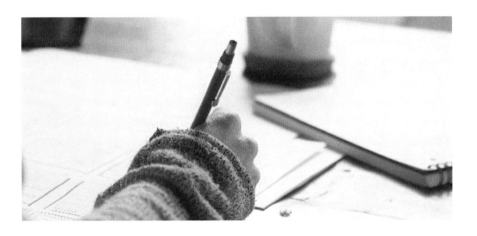

66

"ONE INSURANCE MANDATED PSYCH VISIT BEFORE SURGERY IS NOT ENOUGH TO FIX HEAD SPACE."--DR. V

GET THERAPY TO ADDRESS THE ROOT OF YOUR FEARS AND MIND GAMES.

POST SIDE-BY-SIDE BEFORE AND AFTER PHOTOS ON SOCIAL MEDIA TO DOCUMENT PHOTOGRAPHIC PROOF OF CHANGE.

Self-promote. Celebrate and chronicle your weight-loss progress. Ignore anyone who complains. You aren't doing it for them. You are practicing self-love.

Create healthy eating habits. You become obese only by the foods you eat. Be mindful of what you eat and why. Keep a food log on your phone using an app.

Practice Self Love and affirmations. If you love yourself more than you fear failure, you will do the things necessary to get your health, life and mind back in order.

YOU HAVE ONE LIFE. Resolve to live it in a way that you will not have regrets on your deathday.

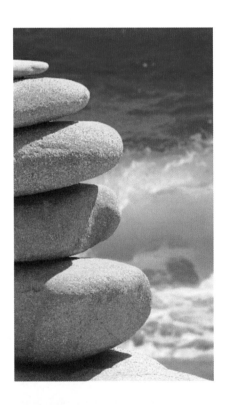

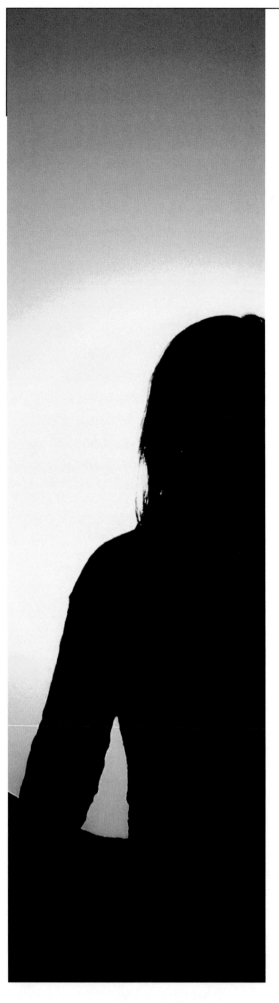

BEGINNER'S MEDITATION EXERCISE

STEP ONE

- Find a comfortable place and remove all distractions. Turn off the phone. Ask people to give you a set amount of time to yourself. Start with just 5 minutes daily and work your way up.

STEP TWO

- Find a comfortable, relaxed position with good posture.
- Close your eyes and focus attention on the self. Your body. Relax any areas that feel tense or tight.

STEP THREE

- Allow yourself to let go of worries and anxieties and other distractions for this set time. Focus instead on measured breathing. Breathe in. Breathe out.

STEP FOUR

- Be kind to yourself. This is not a mystical ceremony. There is no pass or fail in doing it. Meditation is a time to let your brain rest and recharge.
- If your mind wanders to anxieties, insecurities and business of life- gently guide yourself back to mentally observing your breath counts until your meditation session ends.

REPEAT DAILY, SLOWLY EXPAND THE TIME

You can find the science and more detailed exercise tips in my book *Meditate to Lose Weight*.

Gratitude Journal

Date: _____

Write for a minimum of 60 seconds a day

Gratitude Journaling is the easiest yet most important way you can battle the negative mind games. List out all the things you are grateful for, starting each one with the phrase "I am thankful and grateful for _____."

_____

_____

_____

_____

_____

_____

_____

_____

_____

_____

Final Thoughts

Fear has a way of playing with our minds.

But the solution to fear is self love.

In the end we have ONLY one life to live. No do-overs.

So we might as well love ourselves enough to live it now.

Your time is now!

Let go of fear!

Live each day in a way so that you will have no regrets on your deathday.

[1] Dawes AJ, Maggard-Gibbons M, Maher AR, et al. Mental Health Conditions Among Patients Seeking and Undergoing Bariatric SurgeryA Meta-analysis. JAMA. 2016;315(2):150–163. doi:10.1001/jama.2015.18118

[2] Bhatti JA, Nathens AB, Thiruchelvam D, Grantcharov T, Goldstein BI, Redelmeier DA. Self-harm Emergencies After Bariatric SurgeryA Population-Based Cohort Study. JAMA Surg. 2016;151(3):226–232. doi:10.1001/jamasurg.2015.3414

[3] McGrice, M., & Don Paul, K. (2015). Interventions to improve long-term weight loss in patients following bariatric surgery: challenges and solutions. Diabetes, Metabolic Syndrome and Obesity: Targets and Therapy, 8, 263–274. http://doi.org/10.2147/DMSO.S57054

MASTERCLASS 11

15 Ways to Stop Weight Regain

:

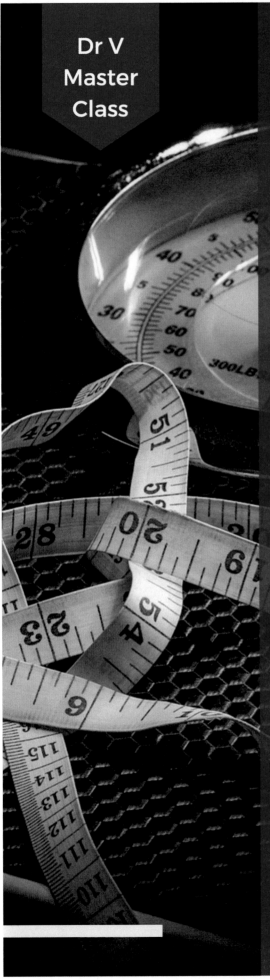

15 WAYS TO STOP WEIGHT REGAIN AFTER WEIGHT LOSS SURGERY

5 Things to Stop Doing
5 Things to Start Doing
5 Things to Start Thinking

Presented by Dr. Duc Vuong

YOU CAN TAKE CONTROL OF YOUR WEIGHT

You made the life-changing decision to have weight loss surgery, and now you are on your way to a new life. Still, the worry that you could regain the weight is ever-present. Or worse, you've actually regained some weight and now are desperate to get it off.

The good news is that you can combat this concern with very simple strategies. However, it will take commitment and dedication on your part.

DECIDE RIGHT NOW THAT YOU WILL COMMIT TO DOING ALL 15 OF THE THINGS SUGGESTED IN THIS DOCUMENT.

Your new health is maintained or broken by a lifetime of habits and choices you make from TODAY onward.

These simple habits will add up to a lifetime of better health, without adding to your budget.

1. STOP SODA

Soda is liquid junk. Made up almost entirely of artificial ingredients, it has absolutely no nutritional value. Even diet soda has an abundance of two of the things you need to take in moderation: sodium and artificial sugar.

We could go over the negative effects on your blood pressure, blood sugar and kidneys; however, for the purpose of this article, we'll stick with **the problem of hidden calories**. It is very easy to lose track of how many of these drinks you consume in a day. At 120 to 300+ calories per 12 oz serving, it will easily negate all your other efforts to be healthier.

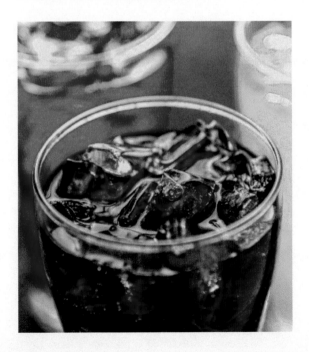

- Steer clear of the 'zero' and 'diet' drinks. They are full of artificial chemicals that affect your body's functions. They provide no nutritional value and can cause leg swelling.
- Drink more water. You body is designed to use water to flush out toxins and keep your body running at its best.
- If you do not like pure water, squeeze some fresh fruit into it or try out some hot or iced spiced herbal teas.
- You can try out samples of various unsweetened drinks at many tea shops like Teavana.
- Soak sliced cucumber and limes in water for 1-5 hours for a cool and refreshing infused drink.
- Make sure to get a minimum of 64oz of water a day to perform at your best.

2. STOP ALCOHOL

Alcohol is very close behind soda in its hidden calories. Even wines are full of simple sugars made during the fermentation process.

Mixed drinks are even worse with sugary syrups and colors to make them appealing. In addition, liver damage is always a serious risk. A small serving of a mixed drink can add hundreds of calories to your daily intake. It does not take much to counteract the progress you made with your new exercise regiment or healthy lunch.

Avoiding alcohol is important for your food intake too. You're more likely to make poor food choices when socializing once you are intoxicated.

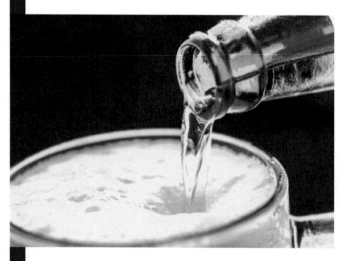
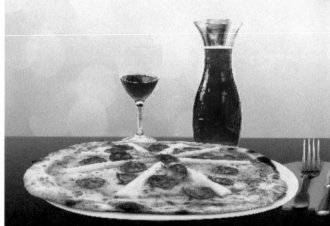

3. Stop Snacking

Remember, it's natural to feel hungry and it's unnatural to feel full.

To lose weight, you must consume fewer calories. To consume fewer calories, you must eat less. In order to eat less, you must allow yourself to get hungry.

Like alcohol, snacking is usually a substitute for something else, whether it's stress, boredom, or emotional. Get to the root cause.

- Drink water when a craving hits. In many cases, our body confuses the first stages of dehydration with hunger. If you think you are hungry, first drink 8oz of water and wait 15 minutes to see if the craving fades.
- Take a walk, read, or enjoy a hobby. When we are bored or under-stimulated, the body will send out hunger signals. Low grade exercise or new mental stimulation often helps turn off the cravings.
- Stop the snacking habit as soon as you can. Limit yourself to only fresh fruit or a handful of nuts. While they are still additional calories that you need to get control of, they are better for you than candy bars, chips, and other snacks. If you're not hungry enough to eat an apple, then you shouldn't be eating.

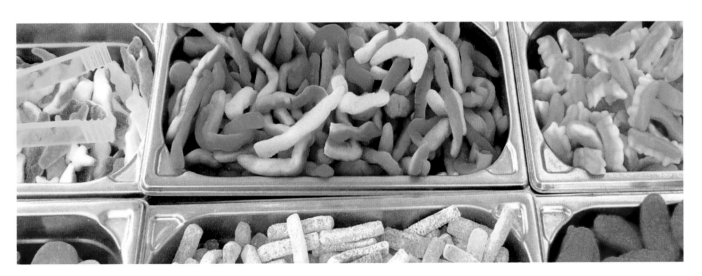

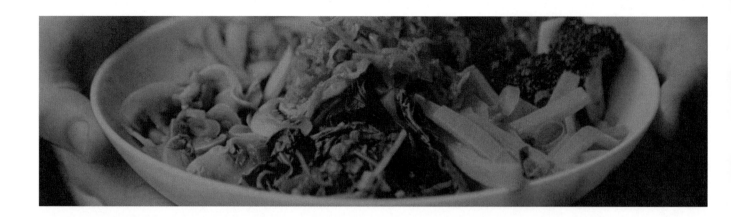

4. STOP BREADS

Breads, muffins and other pastries all quickly add 150+ calories per recommended serving to your meal (before adding butter, jams, or other add-ins). **Bread is nothing more than a vehicle for calories.** Breads also wreak havoc on your blood sugars and are an absolute no-no for diabetics.

Even 'healthy' whole grain and seed breads are guilty of greatly increasing the calories you take in. There are more fulfilling and nutritious whole grains and complex carbs out there to fulfill your needs.

Try out Lettuce and Cabbage wraps for a new and tasty fix. Avoid sandwiches altogether and opt for a big salad (a real salad, not the iceberg 'house salads' people are familiar with). And remember: **PASTA IS A BREAD!**

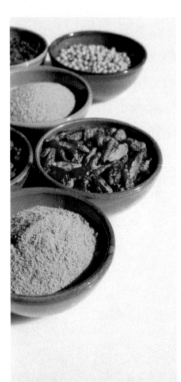

5. STOP CREAMERS AND CONDIMENTS

Coffee creamer adds in extra hidden calories and heart-harming saturated fats with every dose because the volume of coffee consumed probably requires more than just one 40-calorie serving of creamer.

Even the 'fat free' versions of your mayo and creamers have small amounts of bad fat. These harmful fats and untracked calories are not worth the cost of flavoring.

Try coconut milk, spices and herbs, vinaigrette, fruit and other more healthy and flavorful alternatives on foods and drinks.

6. Start Drinking Green Smoothies For Breakfast

When we look at breakfast foods, is it any wonder why obesity rates are at all time highs? A healthier alternative to the typical breakfast of pastries, sugary cereals, or fast food items is a green smoothie.

A green smoothie takes minutes to make, and it provides all the energy you need for your morning routines. You can even cut and freeze most fruits for a week's worth of ingredients.

The leafy greens and fresh fruits are a natural and easily digested source of fiber, vitamins, minerals, antioxidants, and even amino some acids, which is especially important if you've had weight loss surgery. The fruit combinations provide variety and softens the robust flavor of the greens. Check out my green smoothie recipes on Amazon if you need more ideas.

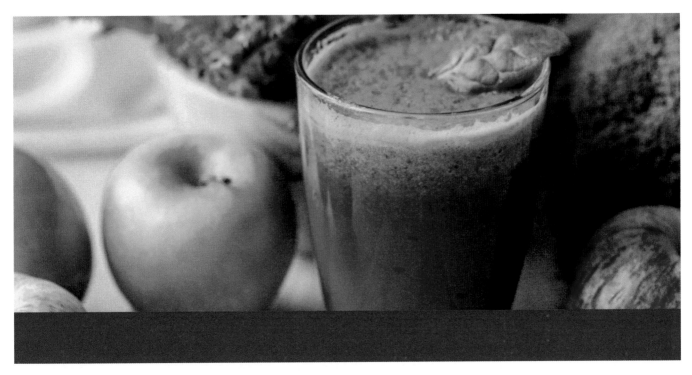

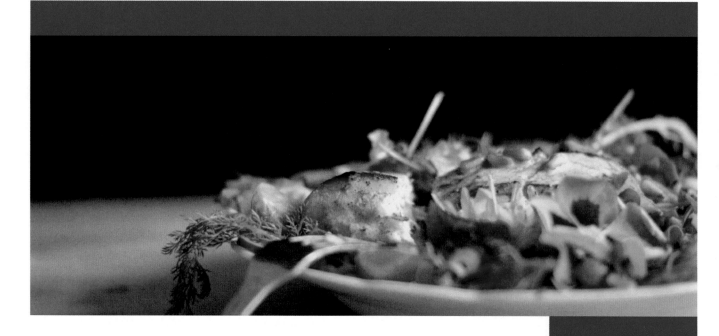

7. START EATING BIG SALADS FOR LUNCH

Not the iceburg lettuce and a scattering of carrots and tomatoes. A proper salad is made up of a variety of toppings and leafy greens--even quinoa, seafood, and fruit toppings.

A salad provides a huge boost in energy and nutrients per calorie. It has great nutrient density. It can be made with baby spinach, sprout mixes, or any other leafy greens as the base. A salad can have cooked ingredients in it like grilled shrimp, beans, sweet potato, quinoa, or wild rice.

When preparing a salad, be careful of fat filled dressings, like Ranch or Thousand Islands. If you need a little dressing, try some fresh salsa, citrus and olive oil, or a nice vinaigrette.

8. START EATING MORE LEAN PROTEINS

I always encourage my patients to get away from red meats entirely, given that so many more plant based alternatives exist.

You can get your nutritional needs entirely from plant based whole foods, even the essential amino acids. In fact, there are several super foods that have all the same proteins and nutrients that we rely on meat for, such as soy and quinoa.

In addition to protein, nuts, seeds, broccoli, beans, and leafy greens also provide a rich assortment of micronutrients and fiber on very few calories per serving. Advances with soy and black beans also make them tasty meat substitutes in various dishes.

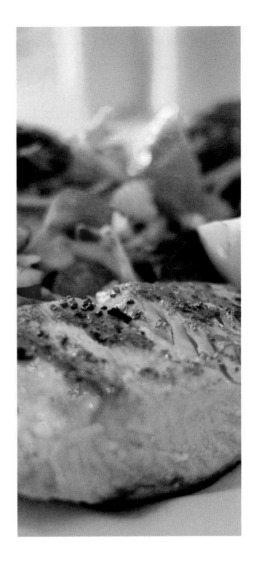

- If you want to keep meat in your menu, you can still make healthier choices. Salmon and other fish are rich in good fats and amino acids.
- Avoid beef and pork as they are high in saturated fats.
- Chicken is not that healthy any more due to the steroids and antibiotics required during mass production.

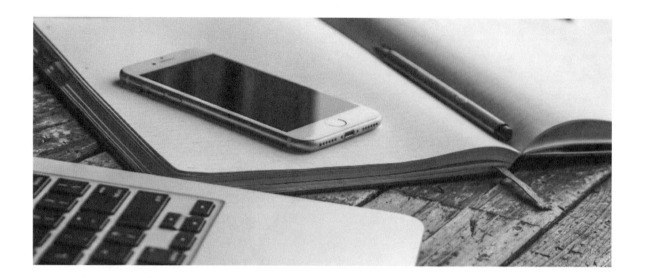

9. Start Food Journaling

The best thing you can do for yourself is to be aware of your eating habits. It is these habits that will make or break your efforts to keep the weight off. However, simply knowing you just drank your third soda or skipped your vegetables today does not have the same impact as seeing it in writing.

There are various apps out there that will help you record what you eat through out the day. Some even come with hints and badges for certain achievements to keep you motivated. If technology is not your thing, a simple notebook is a great tool. Simply write down everything you eat (including drinks and condiments), the date and time, and other notes like known calories, the place, the occasion, and your mood.

As you fill your journal, you will be able to identify eating patterns, such as eating popcorn while watching your favorite tv show or that you drink far more empty calories than you realized. Or perhaps you have a habit of eating unhealthy foods at a specific weekly gathering. You can then tweak these negative patterns to avoid regaining the excess weight.

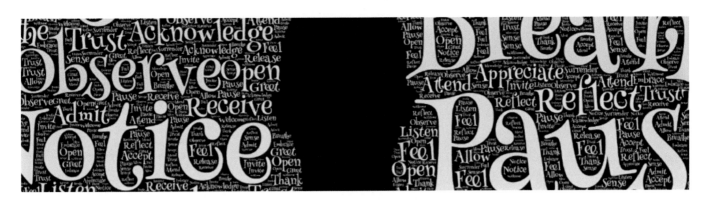

10. **START GRATITUDE JOURNALING**

If you want to immediately impact all areas of your life, then start a gratitude journal. A gratitude journal is a place you spend a part of the day reflecting on good things in your life. Your experiences. Accomplishments. Random acts of kindness. Things that made you smile.

Typically, this is done at the end of the day to break the stress cycle and go to sleep with the positives on your mind. This leads to lower overall stress, raise self awareness, and gain higher perspective.

Start out about 15 minutes before bed and write down 5-10 things that made you happy today and why. It might be a challenge at first, and that is okay. Within a few days, you will start actively looking for these positive things to fill your nightly report. It won't be long before you can list 20 or more things with no effort at all.

When you feel down, frustrated or discouraged pull out your journal and read through it to remind yourself of all the positives in your life. This will help you stay motivated in your journey to good health, and it will help you keep your resolve not to use food as a source of comfort.

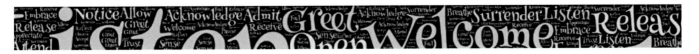

11. THINK: "I AM MORE POWERFUL THAN FOOD"

You are an amazing and complex human being. You have the power to change your habits. You have the power to resist cravings. You have the power to choose healthier habits that fit your new life best.

Food does not have the power to take this away from you. Whenever an urge toward an unhealthy eating choice hits, you have the power to take a step back and reflect on the cost of that choice. You have the power to change your mind. You have the power to make foods accessible or inaccessible in your home. You have the power to refuse to let food dictate your choices. **Always remember you are the one in control, not your cravings.**

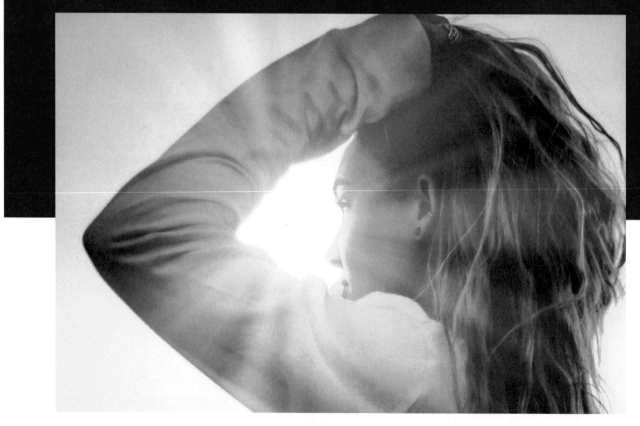

12. THINK: "I CAN BE BETTER"

Look at how far you have already come. You recognized you had a serious problem with your weight, and you took measures to take care of it. This is proof positive in itself that you have the power to change and improve your life.

Now is not the time to rest on your laurels. You can still keep improving. You can learn more about your health. You can change your eating habits. You can learn new skills. No matter how far you've come, there is always a new goal you can reach for to make yourself even better today than yesterday. More importantly, you have the power to learn and improve on mistakes and setbacks.

Falling into a bad habit is not a sign that you are forever destined to live with it. It is a sign you have a habit to replace with a better one. You have the ability and limitless human potential to do exactly that.

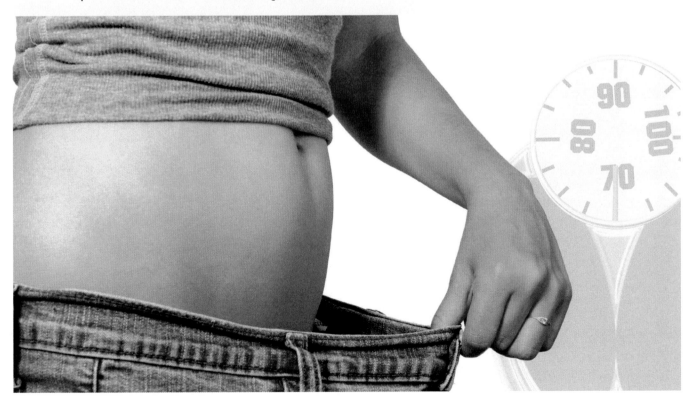

13. THINK: "I DESERVE GOOD HEALTH"

Every human being, including you, has the right to live their lives to their fullest potential. You have the right to strive to be a better person today than you were yesterday.

You have the right to have the good health you need to reach your goals. You deserve to have good health to carry you to your dreams. You are entitled to a long life with your family and loved ones.

As someone who deserves to live this one life to the fullest, it is up to you to make the healthy choices you need to achieve this.

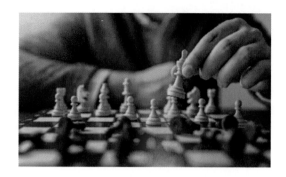

14. THINK: "I CAN LEARN MORE"

We live in a time when just about everything we could want to know is literally at our fingertips.

There are thousands of videos, blogs, books, articles, podcasts and more on just about every topic, all of it easily accessible from a phone, tablet, or computer.

No matter how much you know about your health, there is always something new to learn.

Take a few minutes out if each day to learn a new recipe, a new way to save for your goals, a new life skill, or information that will enhance and enrich your new healthier life.

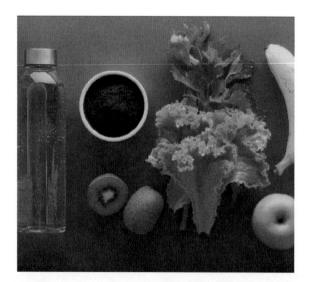

15. THINK: "I DESERVE TO PLACE MYSELF FIRST"

You have one life. No one knows the ins and outs of that life better than you. No one can live that life better than you.

That said, while we ideally want people in our lives to support our decisions, humans as a species are imperfect creatures. There will be times when a friend will urge you to partake of that unhealthy deep fried confection their spouse made. A restaurant will refuse to allow you to substitute those fries or loaded baked potato for a salad. A coworker will say something insensitive about the green smoothie you brought for breakfast.

Temptations to just go with the flow and make those unhealthy choices will come.

It is not your place in life to sacrifice your health for the convenience of others. If someone does not respect your healthier choices, you are not obligated to eat or drink anything that damages your goals.

YOU HAVE EVERY RIGHT TO PLACE YOURSELF FIRST.

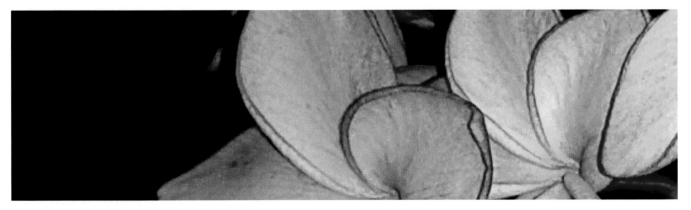

DEDICATE TO DOING THESE 15 HABITS TO PREVENT WEIGHT REGAIN

These tips are all things you can start today and carry with you for a lifetime.

They are practical tools and weapons against the bad habits that contribute to regaining weight after surgery.

If you master them, you will be well on your way to a healthier you!

Dr. Duc Vuong

Dr. Duc Vuong helps people break free from unwanted patterns and limiting beliefs so that they can start over and be more. Although he began his career as an internationally renowned bariatric surgeon, who is the world's leading expert in education for the bariatric patient, his methodologies work for any person in any area of life.

Trained in Western medicine, he blends traditional Eastern teachings with the latest in science and technology. Dr. Vuong was featured in TLC's hit show, 900 Pound Man: Race Against Time, and is currently working on his own weekly television show. He is the author of multiple Amazon best selling books.

Visit **DucVuong.com** to see his online courses

Books
Ultimate Gastric Sleeve Success
Weight Loss Surgery Success: A-Z Tips
Duc-It-Up: 366 Tips
Eating Healthy on a Budget
Eating Healthy For Kids
50 Healthy Green Smoothies
Big-Ass Salads

Get your Dr. V books at Amazon page: www.amazon.com/author/drv
Get your own Dr. V t-shirt at: www.drvgear.com
Talk with Dr. V Live at www.facebook.com/doctorvuong
Get short snippets of wisdom: www.instagram.com/drducvuong

52007065R00109